MAKING SENSE OF MANAGED CARE

Volume I: Building Blocks and Fundamentals

Edited by Kimball Austin Miller, MD, MSHA
and Elaine King Miller, PhD

American College of Physician Executives
Tampa, Florida

Jossey-Bass Publishers
San Francisco, California

ISBN: 0-924674-51-2

Library of Congress Card Number: 97-70473

Printed in the United States of America by Hillsboro Printing, Tampa, Florida

Introduction to Series

In the past decade, the health care delivery system has experienced dramatic changes in both the reimbursement and the administration of services. As these changes are integrated into the current health care system, physicians and health care administrators must not only understand the reasons for the change, but must also quickly respond to the new challenges managed care systems will continue to bring to their practice.

Physicians must quickly and effectively make the transition from traditional fee-for-service practice to managed care practice to compete in today's health care market. The health care professional is well positioned to lead the change to a patient-directed system. Providers are concerned about the heavy emphasis today on issues of cost management and quality analysis, but it is these concepts and techniques that will provide the basis for improved cost accounting and quality assessment measures, which, in turn, will guide a patient-directed system.

The transition to managed care requires physicians and health care administrators to learn as much as possible about the expectations and needs of patients and payers using a variety of managed care models. Only then can physicians continue to be the best advocates for the health care needs of their patients. In addition, health care providers and administrators who integrate delivery system changes into their clinical and administrative decision making will be in the best position to take advantage of the new opportunities that managed care systems can bring to physicians, administrators, and patients.

The series of which this book is a part will allow physicians and health care administrators to educate themselves about the myriad theories and models behind the dramatic shift toward managed care systems, the development of market-driven practices that are responsive to the needs of the many players in the health care system, and the tools necessary to create high-quality and low-cost delivery systems within the managed care framework. It is only through education and participation that health care professionals will be able to continue to be the best advocates for their patients and deliver the highest quality care while remaining competitive in the health care delivery systems market.

Thomas L. Adams, CAE
Executive Vice President and Chief Executive Officer
Medical Group Management Association
Englewood, Colorado

Foreword

Although there are still health care professionals out there who believe that a Maginot Line approach to managed care is the appropriate response, their numbers are dwindling. Most understand that managed care is here to stay—perhaps not in its present form but in a form nevertheless that will continue to transform the delivery and financing of health care services. The key to successfully navigating the sometimes stormy waters of change that managed care has introduced to the health care field will be in understanding managed care and the numerous offspring that it has produced.

It is such understanding that this series of books hopes to cultivate. In Volume I, some of the most creative thinkers in managed care provide a backdrop for issues that will be introduced and expanded upon in later books. If you have decided to start your exploration of managed care with this book, rather than skip to the more complicated and detailed volumes that follow, we congratulate you for your perspicacity, particularly if you are a recent convert to the power and potential of managed care. A grounding in the fundamentals of managed care—its terms, its actors, and its organizational and structural dimensions—is essential to the understanding required.

In this book, you are introduced to the lexicon of managed care, to its essential ingredients and relationships, and to the organizational and structural entities that contain and serve it. A good deal of attention is paid to the move toward integrated delivery systems. Most observers consider managed care and this structural change in the health care system to be partners. Both must be understood. Both must be dealt with.

We are predisposed, of course, but we are confident that you have embarked on the first leg of what will become a magnificent voyage. We look forward to visiting with you again in the final volumes of the book series.

Mark A. Doyne, MD, FACPE
President
American College of Physician Executives
May 1997

Preface

Managed care in its varied forms is rapidly becoming the dominant provider reimbursement format for public and private health care in the United States. Currently, there are few communities or regional health care markets that do not have some form of managed care insurance program, and many markets now have the majority of all care provided under this mechanism. Recent reports regarding the insured marketplace document that two-thirds of employers currently offer health maintenance organization plans and three-quarters offer the option of preferred provider organization plans to their employees. Following the path chosen by commercial payers, many states are actively directing Medicaid recipients into capitated managed care programs, and marketing statistics show a rapid growth in selection of the managed care option by Medicare recipients.

This dramatic and fundamental change in the financing, delivery, and clinical practice of medicine has radically affected provider practice structure, physician interactions with other providers, relationships between physicians and patients, and the day-to-day operations of all health care providers. The major systemwide change has been the transformation of the reimbursement system from a fee-for-service, volume-dependent model to a fixed price per patient (global capitation or per diem/per case payment), risk-sharing model. Managed care thus represents a shift from a profit per unit to a cost per unit philosophy for providers and payers.

This first book in the *Making Sense of Managed Care* series reviews the basic organizational building blocks and theoretical models fundamental to the integrated managed care environment. All health care providers can use this information as a primer to develop their understanding of the history and current status of the managed care universe. The fundamental changes occurring in health care delivery cannot be dismissed as a temporary trend or fad. Building on the financial models, administrative and medical management policies and procedures, and the forecasts of future trends that are discussed by the authors in this book, providers can examine their current positions, determine their strengths, and develop action plans to overcome their vulnerabilities. Our intent is to have providers use this information to orient their professional careers and clinical activities to take full advantage of managed care opportunities.

Unfortunately, time is not on providers' side. All health care providers must rapidly develop a practice style that is service-oriented and perceived to provide health care that is affordable and of high value and quality. Although the exact design of the managed health care delivery system of the future remains cloudy, the key ingredients are coming into focus. The successful health care provider of the next decade will be flexible and responsive to the changing needs, wants, and demands of payers of health care and to the desires of patients. Such providers will be vigilant regarding their environment, ever focused on the health care delivery horizon.

Kimball Austin Miller, MD, MSHA
Denver, Colorado
May 1997

Elaine King Miller, PhD
Fort Collins, Colorado

Table of Contents

Chapter 1 Lexicon of Managed Care Concepts and Terms 1
by Kimball Austin Miller, MD, MSHA, and Elaine King Miller, PhD

Chapter 2 Understanding the Fundamentals of Managed Health Care 17
by Peter R. Kongstvedt, MD, FACP

Chapter 3 Health Maintenance Organizations 47
by Diana Barrett, DBA

Chapter 4 Independent Practice Association Model of Managed Care 63
by Budd N. Shenkin, MD, MAPA

Chapter 5 Overview of Physician Hospital Organizations and Physician Organizations 75
by Eileen Weis, MSHA, and Kimball Austin Miller, MD, MSHA

Chapter 6 Management Service Organizations 91
by Jeffrey R. Hoffman

Chapter 7 Managed Care Contracting Models 101
by David A. Puffer and Kimball Austin Miller, MD, MSHA

Chapter 8 Vertically Asset Integrated Health Care Systems 113
by Thomas L. Kelly

Chapter 9 Virtually Integrated Health Care Systems 125
by Leonard D. Schaeffer and Dana E. McMurtry

Chapter 10 Capstone View: The Integration Paradigm Shift 137
by Kimball Austin Miller, MD, MSHA

Index 143

Table of Contents of Volumes II & III

Volume II: Strategic Positioning

Chapter 1 Economic Issues in Managed Care: Why Health Policy Changes Are About to Ruin Your Life as a Health Care Provider *by Marc J. Roberts, PhD*

Chapter 2 Patient Patients No More: Aging Baby Boomers and Health Care *by Daniel Perry*

Chapter 3 Merger and Acquisitions *by Hobart Collins and Robert C. Bohlmann, FACMPE*

Chapter 4 Capitation *by Timothy F. Harris, FSA, MAAA, and Robert M. Damler, FSA, MAAA*

Chapter 5 Using Patient Satisfaction as a Strategic Weapon *by Elaine King Miller, PhD*

Chapter 6 Medical Care Marketing in the Managed Care World *by Rollie Tillman Jr., MBA, DBA, and Melinda Privette, MD, JD*

Chapter 7 Selecting a Managed Care Plan Partner: Indicators You Can Use *by David E. Vogel, MS*

Chapter 8 Positioning a Health Care Organization Using Value Purchasing Information *by David B. Friend, MD, MBA, and John A. Menefee, PhD*

Chapter 9 Pharmacoeconomics *by Diana I. Brixner, RPh, PhD, Paul Pochtar, RPh, and J. Eric Talbott*

Chapter 10 Information Tools and Managed Care: What You Need to Survive *by Jerome H. Carter, MD, FACP*

Chapter 11 Getting Beyond the Legal Issues in Managed Care *by Donald L. Holmquest, MD, JD*

Chapter 12 Managing Health: Determinants of Clinical Practice *by Kimball Austin Miller, MD, MSHA*

Volume III: Operational Issues and Practical Answers

Chapter 1 Managed Care from the Health Plan Perspective *by Spencer P. Falcon, MD, and Keith C. Kosel, PhD*

Chapter 2 Improving Organizational Performance through Total Quality Management *by John J. Aluise, PhD*

Chapter 3 Organizational Behavior: Tools and Practices for Success in Managed Care Environments *by Elaine King Miller, PhD*

Chapter 4 Cost Control and Practice Management *by David W. Young, DBA*

Chapter 5 Retooling, Restructuring, and Repositioning Medicine to Meet the Consumer Challenge *by Sue Cook and Russell C. Coile Jr.*

Chapter 6 Managed Care Contract Negotiations *by Bruce A. Johnson, JD, MPA*

Chapter 7 Management in Practice: A Case of Risks and Rewards *by Curtis B. McLaughlin, DBA*

Chapter 8 The Role of Guidelines in Successful Managed Care Practice *by Richard Doyle, MD*

Chapter 9 Positive Approaches to Clinical Practice Improvement *by Kathleen Jennison Goonan, MD*

Chapter 10 Measuring Performance of Health Care Providers *by Randall K. Spoeri, PhD, and Robert Futterman, PhD*

Chapter 11 The Role of Patient Satisfaction Surveys in the Assessment of Quality *by David M. Radosevich, PhD*

Chapter 12 Measuring Medical Practice: The Practice Profile *by Vernon B. Hunt, MD MPH*

Chapter 13 Controlling Access: The Cutting Edge Operational Issue in Managed Care *by Kimball Austin Miller, MD, MSHA*

Chapter 1

Lexicon of Managed Care Concepts and Terms

by Kimball Austin Miller, MD, MSHA, and Elaine King Miller, PhD

Successfully initiating and sustaining health care practices and organizations in the managed care environment requires the organizational leadership to carefully analyze potential growth opportunities in its environment and to develop a strategic plan for interventions that are consistent with the organization's purpose and objectives as well as with the demands of the managed care environment. Managed care is a process in which the activities of medical management and control of service demand are imposed on patients and care providers as a condition of their participation in a specific commercial, public sector (Medicaid and Medicare), or employer self-insured health care insurance program. Furthermore, managed care programs result in financial risk shifting partially or totally to providers. It brings organizational and operations management components of systems analysis, accountability/control, and resource management to bear on the health care delivery system.

Until recently, providers directly billed patients on a provider-patient negotiated fee-for-service basis and determined the course of medical treatment through discussions with only patients and close family members. With the initiation of third-party payer insurance, which dramatically increased in mid-century, and the growth of prepaid health maintenance coverage over the past 20 years, an environment conducive to regulation of reimbursement of provider service, forced provider participation in financial risk arrangements, and external controls on patient care management decision making and implementation has emerged. Federal legislation, such as the HMO Act of 1973, added support to corporate initiatives promoting managed care and were conceptually designed to decrease health care costs by controlling utilization of health care resources and provider reimbursement schedules.

Managed health care has increased dramatically during the 60 years since managed care control processes of demand and medical management were first imposed on providers and patients. In 1929, the first prepaid group of a few hundred families was formed in Elk City, Oklahoma, by a rural farmers' cooperative. The shareholder-owned health plan paid physician members on a discounted medical care rate schedule from annual dues paid by enrollees. This pioneer program was quickly followed by well-known prepaid health maintenance organization (HMO) programs, such as Group Health Association of Washington in 1937, Kaiser-Permanente Medical Care in 1942, and Group Health Cooperative of Puget Sound in 1947.

These prepaid managed care health plans initiated monumental change in health care financing by shifting payers, providers, and patients from a fee-for-service billing model to a prepaid per capita payment for medical treatment. Total enrollment in managed care plans (HMOs, preferred provider organizations (PPOs), and exclusive provider organizations (EPOs)) now exceeds 155 million members. Managed care is the predominant form of health care coverage nationally. Currently, more than 20 percent of all patients have HMO insurance and more than 35 percent have PPO/EPO coverage. Metropolitan enrollment is the major source of HMO membership, with more than 90 percent of all HMO enrollees residing in metropolitan markets. The average HMO market penetration is 26 percent in large markets (more than 1 million population), 17 percent in medium markets (250,000-999,999 population), and 12 percent in small markets (fewer than 250,000 population).[1,2]

In 1996, with regard to the 669 operational HMO plans then in existence, 65 percent were independent practice association (IPA) type plans, 25 percent were network or group model plans, and 10 percent were employed physician staff models. The tax status for these HMO plans is 70 percent for profit and 30 percent not-for-profit. The nation's 46 HMO chains covered 83 percent of all HMO enrollees. Medical loss ratios were 84 percent for large HMOs and 79 percent for small plans, with 83 percent of all HMO plans achieving profitability. Surveys have documented that capitation is the most common method (62 percent) of physician reimbursement by HMOs and that the typical health plan contracts with an average of 1,800 physicians.[2-6]

Analysis of the PPO and EPO industry in mid-1995 indicates there were 763 operational PPO/EPO programs with 67 million PPO and 10 million EPO enrollees. Current estimates predict that 1996 year-end data will document PPO/EPO membership reaching slightly more than 91 million members. The typical PPO provided payers of health care with savings through access to a panel of discounted fee-for-service providers, utilization review, quality assurance, claims processing, and drug formularies. The average PPO contracted with 4,985 physicians and 83 hospitals. Forty-five percent of PPOs were owned by insurance companies, with the next largest groups being health care provider organizations and independent investors. Overall, 81 percent of operational PPOs reported a profit or break-even status.[7,8]

Because a PPO/EPO typically takes no insurance risk and only facilitates access to a panel of discounted fee providers and performs medical management activities, it is not surprising that the typical source of eligible members is 58 percent through health insurance companies, 23 percent through third-party administrators, and 19 percent through contracts with self-insured employers.[7] This discounted fee managed care model usually pays preferred providers 15-20 percent and exclusive providers 20-25 percent less than community fees for services to enrolled members.

However, unlike the capitated, closed-panel managed care model, the PPO delivery format will usually reimburse members for services provided by nonpreferred or exclusive providers, but only at the discounted rate, with the balance being the responsibility of the enrollee. The resource utilization aspects of PPO / EPO managed care are based on the use of provider withholds and medical management activities.

All insurance companies, either indemnity entities (also by historical coincidence first started in 1929) or managed care intermediaries (MCI), assume responsibility for providing a complete spectrum of medical care to a select membership at a predetermined premium. The issue that differentiates managed care intermediaries from indemnity insurers is the shifting of some or all financial risk to providers. If hospital and physician members of the provider delivery group (jointly, as a physician hospital organization (PHO), partnership health organization, or integrated delivery system (IDS), or separately, as a contractually bound hospital and physician organization (PO)/independent practice association) incur expenses that are greater than the actuarially agreed upon revenue, the deficit is in part or fully the responsibility of providers (figure 1, below).

Figure 1. Managed Care Risk Food Chain

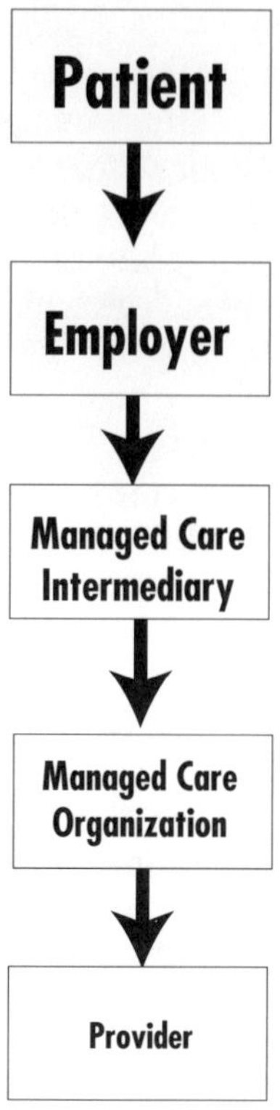

This shift from the provider no-risk model of traditional fee-for-service reimbursement, where providers had no formal incentive to reduce health care utilization and possibly were encouraged to overutilize, to one of shared risk (capitation, discounted fee for service with withholds) formed the basis for the initiation of demand management and other medical management activities. These managed care programs monitor providers for overutilization and at the same time prevent possible underutilization caused by prepayment. The programs monitor service and clinical outcome measures to determine the appropriate utilization guidelines for the health plan. All the tools and activities used by a medical management program must affect and measure both cost and quality.

Demand management is an access control process in which patient needs are matched with the most cost-efficient type and site of service delivery. For example, demand management techniques determine the medical delivery parameters for an acute illness encounter by choosing the appropriate provider (registered nurse, advanced practice nurse, generalist physician, or secondary care specialist) and the location of the encounter (phone triage/advice, home visit, office visit, urgent care visit, emergency department visit, or hospitalization). The goal of demand management is matching provider resources with the member's needs and wants while promoting long-term quality of care and cost efficiency. To encourage patients to accept demand management policies, various coinsurance and copayment mechanisms are implemented by the health plan administration.

Medical management is traditionally composed of clinical and administrative activities. The clinical management processes include provider credentialing/selection, utilization management (prior authorization, certification for claims adjudication, concurrent review, case and disease management, utilization review, second opinion, and referral management), quality assurance, formulary management, health promotion, and outcome measurement. The administrative components of medical management are relationship management, demand management (using clinical protocols and algorithms), and grievance abatement and resolution. These activities are the direct responsibility of the managed care intermediary (the entity with state insurance license) but can be performed as a joint effort with the managed care organization with the sharing of risk. The managed care process is rooted in provider credentialing/selection, utilization management, and quality assurance (peer review, continuous quality improvement programs, and clinical practice guidelines). Because a managed care organization (MCO) is a group of providers organized to provide the full spectrum of health care, they are an ideal format for performing the managed care process.

All managed care processes focus their energy and efforts on preventing under- or overutilization of medical resources, promoting high-quality care based on outcome measurement, and encouraging cost-efficient allocation of resources across the spectrum of clinical care delivery. Integrated health maintenance organizations merge the delivery and financing of care into one system and can be viewed as a combination of an MCI and an MCO (figure 2, page 5). These entities can vary in structure from the open-format model, with the relationship between the health plan (managed care intermediary) and individual providers, to network alliances between the health plan and provider groups, to fully vertically integrated models with (staff-model HMO) or without (virtually or contractually bound model) merging of assets and centralized control. These united entities have the potential because of their formal or functional integrated status to be economically most efficient. Because of their integration, they have the ability to innovatively and strategically plan for resource allocation (human, physical plant, financial, and technical) across the entire insurer-provider spectrum.

Figure 2. HMO Models

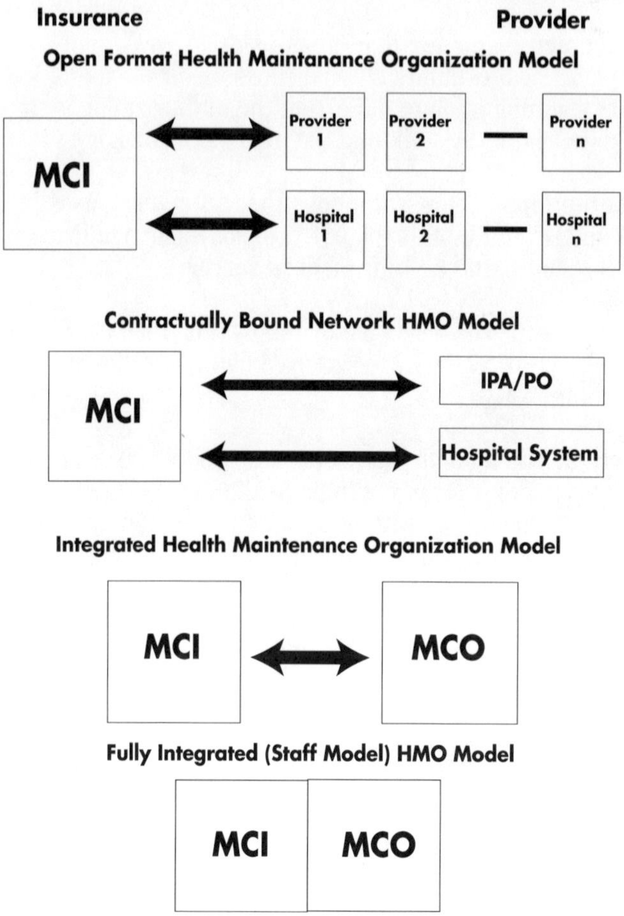

Because PPOs and EPOs are only brokers of panels of providers willing to accept discounted fee-for-service reimbursement and implement only selected medical management methodologies, they are unable to use the integrated approach to planning and resource allocation. Because the integrated planning approach of health care resource utilization is theoretically most economically efficient in the allocation of resources, many health care planners see PPOs as a transition model from the indemnity insurance-independent provider model to a resource integrated nationally or regionally organized but community sensitive HMO delivery system.

In any growing field of expertise or management endeavor, the new group of professionals develop its own language patterns and sets of definitions to define its activities and functions. Managed care as a subset of the health care industry has been no different. As a foundation for readers of this series of books, the following glossary of terms and listing of acronyms and initialisms is provided.[9-12]

Accrual. The amount of money that is set aside to cover expenses or costs. The accrual is the plan's best estimate of what those medical expenses are and is actuarially based on a combination of data from the authorization system, demographic assumptions, the claims system, and the plan's prior history.

Actuarial Assumptions. The assumptions that an actuary uses in calculating the expected costs and revenues of the plan. Examples include utilization rates, age and gender mix of enrollees, and cost for medical services.

Administrative Costs. The costs incurred by the managed care intermediary (insurance company) for claims processing, billing, enrollment, member services, advertising, and the like.

Adverse Selection. The tendency of people with poorer health or with expectations of health problems to apply for or continue health care coverage to a greater degree than people in better health or with expectations of better health. This selection is partially responsible for indemnity insurance costs' being higher than HMO costs.

Age/Gender Factor. A measurement used in actuarial underwriting that uses the age and gender risk of medical costs of one population relative to another population.

Ambulatory Patient Grouping. A patient classification system that categorizes patient outpatient visits to determine reimbursement. In this system, the provider is paid a fixed fee for the patient visit regardless of the resources used during the visit.

Balance Billing. The provider practice of billing a patient for all charges not paid for by the insurance plan. Managed care plans generally prohibit providers from balance billing except for allowed copayments, coinsurance, and deductibles.

Benefit Package. A collection of specific services that the managed care health plan is obligated to provide under terms of its contract with members.

Business Health Coalition. Groups of employers that seek to control health care costs while ensuring quality by aggressively negotiating price on a fixed health benefit package and demanding data on quality and outcomes.

Capitation. A method of payment, frequently employed by HMOs, in which doctors or hospitals are paid a negotiated flat fee for each person to whom they are assigned, regardless of how many services any individual consumes. The object is to shift risk for controlling resource utilization to the service provider. Payment amount is varied by age/gender and is usually expressed in units of per member per month (PMPM).

Carve-Out. A decision by a managed care intermediary to purchase separately a specific group of services that are a portion of the full spectrum of health care from a specialized vendor. For example, an MCI may "carve-out" behavioral health benefits to a specialized vendor.

Case Management. A method of managing the provision of health care to members with chronic, catastrophic, or high-cost medical conditions across the full spectrum of health care delivery. The goal is to coordinate the care to improve continuity and quality of care and to lower costs. Case management generally is a function of the utilization management department.

Closed-Panel Model. A managed care plan that contracts with managed care organizations or a closely affiliated physician group and a hospital on an exclusive basis for services. Patients are required to see physicians on this panel.

Coinsurance. A provision in a member's coverage that limits the amount of coverage by the plan to a certain percentage, commonly 80 percent, of charges. Any additional costs are paid by the member out of pocket.

Community Health Management Information System. An electronic interchange system that links health care purchasers, providers, and payers.

Community Rating. A rating methodology requiring managed care intermediaries to charge the same amount of money per member for all members in the plan. Community rating does allow for variability by allowing the HMO to factor in differences for age, sex, mix (average contract size), and industry factors.

Concurrent Review. Utilization management process of daily evaluation of hospitalized patients using national resource utilization standards that determines medical necessity and appropriateness of service.

Copayment. That portion of a claim or medical expense that a member must pay out of pocket. Usually a fixed amount, such as $5 or $10.

CPT-4. *Current Procedural Terminology, 4th edition.* A set of five-digit codes that apply to medical services and are used for billing by professionals.

Credentialing. Primary source verification of the documentation of professional providers. Such documentation includes, at a minimum, licensure, medical diploma, residency certificates, board certifications, evidence of malpractice insurance, and malpractice history. The process usually follows NCQA guidelines.

Deductible. That portion of a patient's health care expenses that must be paid out of pocket before any insurance coverage applies, commonly $100 to $300 per benefit year.

Demand Management. Process to match patient needs with high-quality, cost-efficient settings while encouraging member self-care.

Direct Contracting Option. A proposal that would allow doctor and hospital networks to directly contract with Medicare.

Discounted Fee for Service. A financial reimbursement method whereby a provider agrees to provide services on a fee-for-service basis, but with the fees discounted by a certain percentage from the provider's usual charges.

DRG. Diagnosis-related groups. A statistical system of classifying any inpatient stay into disease or injury groups for purposes of payment.

Echo Analysis. A decision-making model that combines economic, clinical, and humanistic outcomes analysis to determine the therapeutic value of a medical intervention.

EDI. Electronic data exchange. Computer-to-computer exchange of financial or other information.

EPMPY. Encounters per member per year.

EPO. Exclusive provider organization. An EPO is similar to a PPO, in that it often uses primary care physicians as gatekeepers, often capitates providers, has a limited provider panel, and uses a utilization management system. It is referred to as exclusive because the member must remain within a limited network (smaller than a PPO) to receive benefits.

ERISA. Employee Retirement Income Security Act. A federal law that allows companies to have self-funded health plans that can directly contract with integrated health care organizations or provider groups. One provision also allows the company to avoid complying with state-mandated benefits requirements and paying state premium insurance rates.

Evaluation and Management Services (E/M). Patient evaluation and management functions performed during physician office visits, outpatient visits, and hospital visits or consultations. They consist of taking a patient history, performing a patient examination, and cognitive medical decision-making.

Fee-for-Service Reimbursement. The traditional health care payment system in which providers receive payment of billed charges.

Fee Schedule. A listing of the maximum fees that a health plan will pay for services, based on CPT billing codes.

Formulary. A listing of drugs that a physician may prescribe. The physician is required to use only formulary drugs unless there is a valid medical reason to use a nonformulary drug.

Gatekeeper/Gate Opener. A primary care provider who coordinates and authorizes all care for plan members from providers except in true emergencies.

Group Model. A type of HMO that contracts with a medical group for the provision of health care services to its members.

HCFA-1500. The universal claim form used by professionals to bill health insurance carriers for services.

HEDIS (Health Plan Employer Data and Information Set). A list of NCQA-determined indicators of health plan performance. The indicators are divided into five categories: quality, enrollee access and satisfaction, utilization factors, finance, and descriptive information on health plan management.

Health Care Financing Administration (HCFA). Agency within the Department of Health and Human Services that administers the Medicare program. HCFA is responsible for overseeing Medicare payment regulations.

Health Status Questionnaire. A multiple-choice, self-administered patient questionnaire used to determine patients' perceptions of their health and functional status.

HMO. Health maintenance organization. An HMO provides health care to voluntarily enrolled members in return for a preset amount of money paid on a PMPM basis. The health plan places at least some of the providers at risk for medical expenses and utilizes primary care physicians as coordinators of the members care. HMOs combine delivery and financing of care in one system.

Horizontal Integration. A descriptive management term applied to organizations that involve the acquisition of or contracting between two or more competitors who provide similar types of health care services.

ICD-9-CM. *International Classification of Diseases, 9th Edition,* clinical modification. Classification of disease by diagnosis code of 6-digit numbers.

IDS. Integrated delivery system. A managed care organization in which usually all physicians are employed, and hospital and practice assets are merged into one business entity.

IPA. Independent practice association. An organization that has a contract with a managed care plan to deliver services to plan members for a fixed total fee. The IPA, in turn, contracts with individual providers to provide services on either a capitation or a fee-for-service basis.

ISN. Integrated service network. A contractually bound network of providers that provide the full spectrum of health services without merging of assets.

Indemnity Plan. An insurance program in which the insured member is reimbursed for all covered expenses by the insurance company.

Integration Model. Formal integration is the development of a health care delivery system with the transfer of all assets and management control to the combined entity. Virtual integration is also a vertically oriented health care delivery network, but participants are contractually bound and there is limited asset transfer.

JCAHO. Joint Commission on Accreditation of Healthcare Organizations. A private, not-for-profit organization that evaluates and accredits hospitals and other health care organizations.

Loss Ratio. The ratio of costs incurred for health care services and the premium. Also sometimes called medical loss ratio.

Managed Care. A system of health care delivery that tries to manage the costs, the quality, and the quantity of health care and access to that care.

MCI. Managed care intermediary. A business entity with a state license to sell managed care insurance to employers and state agencies. Also called managed care plan or managed care health plan.

MCO. Managed care organization. A group of providers organized to provide the full spectrum of health care (PHO/IDS).

Medical Loss Ratio. The ratio of the cost to deliver medical care and the amount of money that is taken in by a plan. If payment rates are too low, the ratio may be high, even though the actual cost of delivering care is not really out of line.

MIS. Management information systems. The term for the computer hardware and software that provides administrative, financial, and medical management information.

NCQA. National Committee for Quality Assurance. A not-for-profit organization that performs quality-oriented accreditation reviews on managed care organizations.

Network Model. A type of HMO that contracts with multiple physician groups to deliver health care to members.

Nonparticipating Physician (Nonpar). A physician who has elected not to sign a participation agreement with the managed care entity. Therefore, the provider is not listed in MCO or MCI directories.

Open-Format Model. A type of HMO that contracts with multiple individual physicians and hospitals to deliver care.

Outcome Measure. An assessment that objectively evaluates the effects and results of treatment for a particular disease.

Participating Physician (Par). A physician who has signed a managed care participation agreement, which binds the physician to accept a set capitation or fee schedule on all member claims within the calendar year.

PCN. Primary care network. A grouping of health providers (physicians, hospitals, pharmacies, psychologist, ambulatory care facilities, etc.) that work as an integrated organization to provide health care services to a select group of health plan members.

PCP. Primary care provider. Generally applies to internists, pediatricians, family physicians, general practitioners, and advanced practice nurses.

Peer Review. Evaluation by professionals with training similar to that of the provider of the medical service of health care provided to a managed care enrollee.

Per Diem Reimbursement. Reimbursement to an institution, usually a hospital, based on a set rate per day rather than on charges.

Pharmacoeconomics. The description and analysis of the costs abd consequences of pharmaceuticals and pharmaceutical services and their impact on individuals, health systems, and society.

PHO. Physician hospital organization. These organizations bond hospitals and physicians into one entity, frequently developed to negotiate and contract with managed care plans.

PMPM. Per member per month. Specifically applies to a revenue or a cost for each enrolled member each month.

PO. Physician Organization. Physicians jointly market their services to managed care intermediaries.

POS. Point of service. A health insurance rider that allows plan members to obtain services outside of the defined plan provider network without referral from their primary care providers.

PPO. Preferred provider organization. A plan that contracts with independent providers at a discounted rate for services. The panel is limited in size and usually has some aspects of medical management. Members must see PPO panel members to get the full discounted benefit.

Practice Guidelines. Statements on medical practice that assist physicians and patients in making decisions about appropriate health care for a specific diagnosis.

Prior Authorization. Process of obtaining certification or authorization from a health plan for routine hospital admissions, specific outpatient activities, and referrals to secondary care specialists and subspecialists.

Provider. Any professional who delivers direct unsupervised care (e.g., allopathic physician, osteopathic physician, or advanced practice nurse) or any health care entity where the services are performed (e.g., hospital, skilled nursing facility, ambulatory surgery facility, or community health center).

PSP. Primary specialist provider. Generally an internal medicine or pediatric specialist or subspecialist who provides primary care and single disease care to selected health plan members.

Quality Assurance. The process of auditing medical care provided to members. Uses provider peer review, practice guidelines, and process improvement policies and procedures.

Reinsurance. A type of protection purchased by managed care intermediaries and managed care organizations from specialized insurance companies. Typical forms of reinsurance risk coverage include individual member stop loss, aggregate group stop loss, and insolvency protection.

Relationship Management. A process to service the needs and wants of providers and the education of providers and their office staffs regarding health plan policies and procedures. Also know as provider relations/services.

Relative Value Unit (RVU). Basic element of measure for RBRVS. Each service is assigned relative value units for physician work, practice expenses, and professional liability insurance. The three units together are the relative value of the service.

RBRVS. Resource-based relative value scale. A relative value scale developed by a Harvard research team that assigns values to physician services on the basis of resource costs of providing those services. Relative value units are modified to reflect local cost variations by multiplying them by geographic practice cost index values established for each region and then by federally determined dollar amounts for the units.

Self-Insured Plan. A health plan in which the risk for medical costs is assumed by the company rather than an insurance company or managed care plan.

Staff Model. A type of HMO that employs providers directly. Providers see members in the plan's own outpatient and inpatient facilities. This is a fully asset integrated system.

Stop Loss. An arrangement between a managed care company and a reinsurer whereby patient expenses are limited either in terms of overall loss for all members or by limiting the loss on a individual member.

TPA. Third-party administrator. A firm that performs administrative functions (e.g., claims processing and membership services).

TQM. Total quality management. An operations management technique using all employees to define production/service processes and improve output quality and cost effectiveness.

Telemedicine. Technology that supports real-time, two-way exchange of medical information between distant points.

UB-92. The common claim form used by hospitals to bill for services.

UCR. Usual, customary, or reasonable. A method of profiling prevailing fees in an area.

Unbundling/Bundling. Separation or aggregation of portions of a specific group of medical services.

Unmarried/Married. The relationship between a PO or an IPA and a hospital system that relates to the nonexclusivity/exclusivity of the contract between the two business entities.

Utilization Management. The process of monitoring resource usage. Composed of prior authorization, certification for claims adjudication, concurrent review, case management, disease management, utilization review, and referral management.

Utilization Review. A formal assessment conducted by professional personnel of medical necessity and usage of medical care resources for a member that looks across the entire health care delivery spectrum.

Value. A function of both the cost and the quality of a product or service.

Vertical Integration. A descriptive management term applied to organizations that involves the acquisition of or contracting with health care entities at different levels in the health care delivery system (e.g., tertiary care hospital and physician office).

Withhold. The "at risk" portion of a claim that is deducted by the MCI or MCO prior to payment to the provider. Only when specific utilization goals are achieved is the "at risk" portion paid to the provider.

Figure 3. Effect of Managed Care on Providers

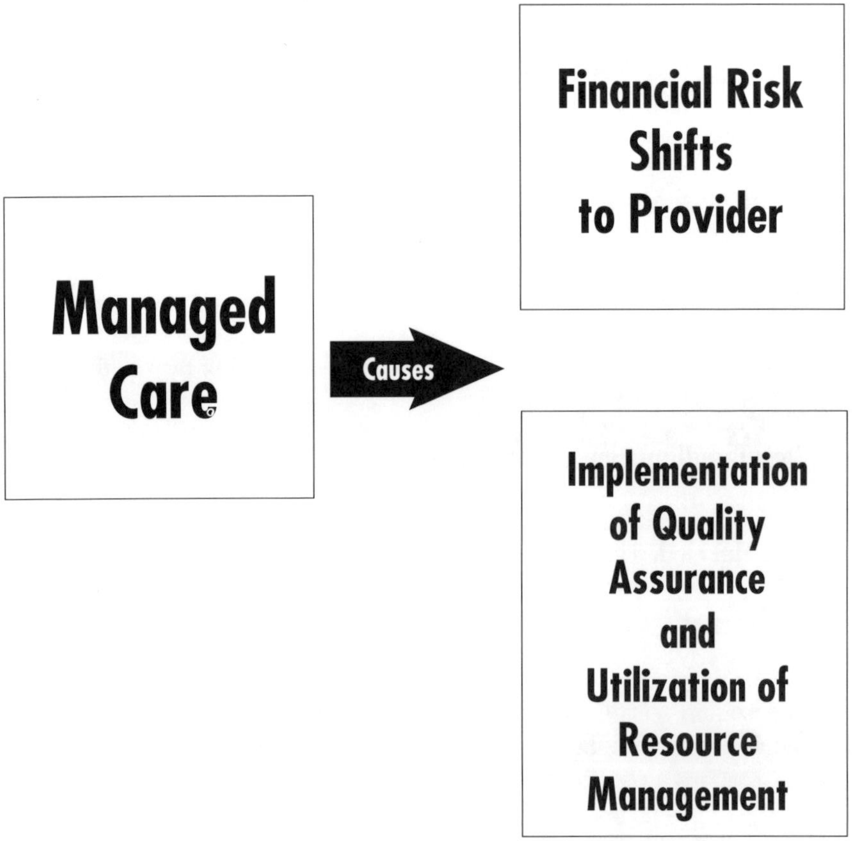

The terms and abbreviation listed above use traditionally accepted definitions for the managed care industry. However, there has been a blurring of many terms as the industry matures and as products are merged and modified to fill market niches and demands. Specifically, the term, managed care organization, is used nationally to mean varied organizational entity types, including HMOs, state-licensed managed care intermediaries, and integrated provider organizations. In this series, an attempt has been made to be more specific with this term. Managed care organization is used to identify an organization that comprises various providers (physician, hospital, advance practice nurse, pharmacy, home health, etc.), is integrated operationally, and has the ability to accept and manage member care and financial risk. This risk can be accepted directly from employers and business coalitions or from affiliated or unaffiliated managed care intermediaries.

In summary, heath care delivery is in dramatic change, and the concept of managed care for physicians and all health care professionals can best be described as a cause-and-effect relationship (figure 3, page 14). Providers and the managed care industry will succeed when they combine their knowledge and skills to develop and implement communitywide health care delivery programs that promote high-quality care at reasonable cost. In addition to quality safeguards, successful provider- or insurer-owned plans will have greater flexibility in providing out-of-network care, the option of self referral to selected specialists, easy access to urgent care and health promotion services, and increased clarity of plan benefits and restrictions. All providers must understand that utilization decisions and quality determinations are still under provider influence and that with risk comes the potential for rewards.

References

1. "Local Health Plans Could Top Big HMOs in '97." *American Medical News* 40(3):3,28, Jan. 20, 1997.
2. "Industry Insights." *Managed Care Outlook* 10(1):4, Jan. 10, 1997.
3. *Managed Care Digest–Integrated Health Systems Digest.* Kansas City, Mo.: Hoechst Marion Roussel, 1996.
4. *The Competitive Edge Regional Market Analysis 6.2.* Minneapolis, Minn.: InterStudy, 1996.
5. *Managed Care Digest–HMO Editions.* Kansas City, Mo.: Marion Merrell Dow, Inc., 1995.
6. *Managed Care Digest–HMO-PO Digest.* Kansas City, Mo.: Hoechst Marion Roussel, 1996.
7. *Managed Care Digest–PPO Edition.* Kansas City, Mo.: Marion Merrell Dow, Inc., 1995.
8. Gerber, P., and Bijlefeld, M. "What's Ahead for Managed Care in 1997." *Physicians Management* 37(1):36, Jan. 1997.
9. "Reform." *American Medical News,* July 6, 1992, pp. 25-32.
10. Kongstvedt, P. *The Managed Care Handbook.* Gaithersburg, Md.: Aspen Publications, 1993.
11. Slee, V. *Health Care Terms.* Ann Arbor, Mich." Tringa Press, 1986.
12. *The Language of Managed Care.* Minnetonka, Minn.: United Healthcare Corp., 1994.

Bibliography

Anthony, R., and Young, D. *Management Control in Nonprofit Organizations.* Burr Ridge, Ill.: Irwin, 1994.

Carson, K., and others. *Management of Healthcare Organizations.* Cincinnati, Ohio: South-Western College Publishing, 1995.

Duncan, W., and others. *Strategic Management of Health Care Organizations, Second Edition.* Cambridge, Mass.: Blackwell Publishers, 1995.

Hammon, J., Editor. *Fundamentals of Medical Management.* Tampa, Fla.: American College of Physician Executives, 1993.

Harris, J. *Strategic Health Management.* San Francisco, Calif.: Jossey-Bass Publishers, 1994.

Lathrop, J. *Restructuring Health Care.* San Francisco, Calif.: Jossey-Bass Publishers, 1993.

Wirth, T., and Allcorn, S. *Creating New Hospital-Physician Collaboration.* Chicago, Ill.: Health Administration Press, 1993.

Kimball Austin Miller, MD, MSHA, is Adjunct Professor of Business Administration, Arizona State University, College of Business, Department of Health Administration and Policy, Tempe, Arizona, and Adjunct Associate Professor of Medicine, University of Oklahoma, College of Medicine, Department of Internal Medicine, Tulsa, Oklahoma. Elaine King Miller, PhD, is Associate Professor of Management, Colorado State University, College of Business, Department of Management, Fort Collins, Colorado. She is a member of the AMA/AAMC Liaison Committee on Medical Education, Washington, D.C.

Chapter 2

Understanding the Fundamentals of Managed Health Care*

by Peter R. Kongstvedt, MD, FACP

Introduction

What is managed health care? Any simple answer would miss the very real forces at work in the health care industry today that have led to the evolution of managed health care. It would likewise miss the substantial positive contributions managed health care has made to the American health care system as we struggle to balance the three key elements of health care—access, cost, and quality.

There are many who believe that unrestrained fee-for-service medicine has led to inappropriately high utilization and is therefore the root cause of our health care cost crisis. While there is merit in the argument, it is simplistic. Health care costs have risen in the past decades at an alarming rate for a multiplicity of reasons, not because of just one reimbursement model—rapidly developing (and usually expensive) technology, cost shifting by providers to pay for care rendered to patients who either cannot pay or are covered by systems that do not pay the full cost of care, shifting demographics as our population ages, high expectations for long and healthy lives, the current legal environment leading to defensive medicine, administrative costs related to the care that is delivered, wide variations in efficiencies and quality of care that is rendered by all types of providers (professional and institutional), serious inequities and variations in incomes between all types of providers (regardless of efficiency or quality), and myriad other reasons. While health care costs have recently slowed, there is no guarantee that they will remain under control, because these forces remain alive today.

The growth of managed care is undeniable and is a one-way phenomenon, as illustrated in figure 1, page 18. These rapid growth rates will continue to accelerate as the public sector moves heavily into managed care and as indemnity insurance continues to dwindle.

---

* Parts of this chapter originally appeared as Chapter 34 in *Health Care Administration*, Wolper, L., Editor, Aspen Publishing, Gaithersburg, Md., 1995; used with permission.

Figure 1. U.S. Insurance Distribution

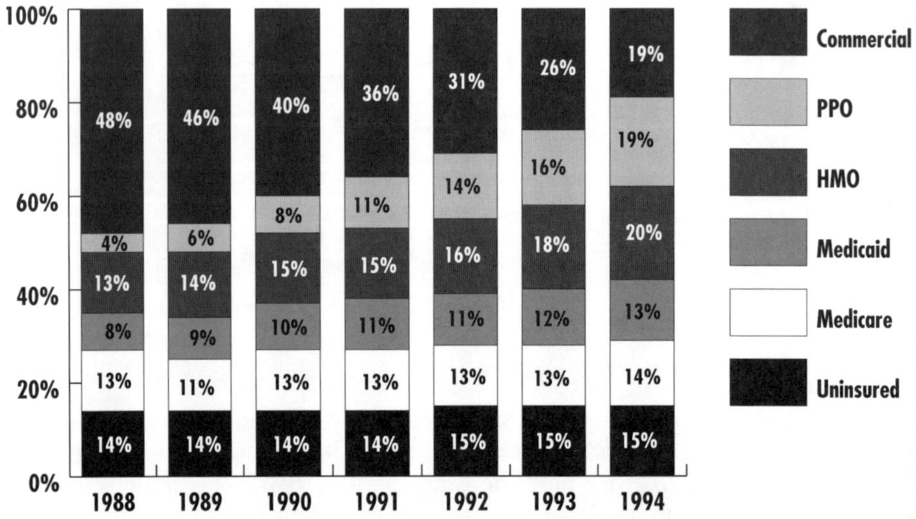

Sources: AAHP (formerly GHAA/AMCRA), Interstudy, Dept. of Commerce, Hoechst Marion Roussel, 1995.

As this chapter is being written, debate over health reform at both the state and federal levels is occurring, and many states have already adopted their own versions of health reform. Reform of the public sector, especially Medicaid, has progressed rapidly. If and when serious health reform is implemented on a broader scale, it is possible that some of the issues presented in this chapter will be rendered inaccurate or even irrelevant, but the concept of managed health care figures prominently in most reform proposals.

The term "member" in this chapter applies to an individual who is insured. The term member may be used interchangeably with the term "patient" (although clearly one may be a member, receive no medical services, and thus not be the patient of any provider, a concept important to actuaries when they calculate risk). A "subscriber" is the individual who actually has the insurance contract; subscriber's dependents receive insurance by virtue of that same contract. Both subscribers and their dependents are considered members. The term "provider" applies to any person or institution that provides medical care. Provider most often refers to a professional (e.g., a physician) but may be used more broadly. Finally, the term "plan" refers to the managed care organization that provides the insurance coverage and manages the delivery system.

Definition of Managed Health Care

Managed health care, or managed care, is an approach to managing both the quality and the cost of medical care. In the current environment, there really is no single definition of managed health care; it is a term applied to a wide variety of systems. In general, there are at least two elements common to managed health care systems: some type of authorization system and some level of restriction on a member's choice of providers. The authorization system may be minimal, such a simple hospital precertification requirement, or it may be comprehensive, such as a primary care physician (PCP) "gatekeeper" model. The restriction on choice of provider may be minimal, such as a minor increase in coinsurance to see an out-of-network provider in a preferred provider organization (PPO), or it may be strict, such as a highly restrictive health maintenance organization (HMO). This chapter will focus on managed care as defined through benefit plan design and operations.

Managed care may be thought of as a continuum of models:

- Indemnity with precertification, mandatory second opinion, and large-case management.
- Service plan with precertification, mandatory second opinion, and large case management.
- Preferred provider organization (PPO)
- Point-of-service (POS)
- "Open-access" health maintenance organization (HMO)
- Traditional HMO
    - Open panel
        - Individual practice association (IPA)
        - Direct contract
    - Network model
    - Closed-panel HMO
        - Group model
        - Staff model

As models move down the continuum, certain changes occur:

- Elements of control over health care delivery become tighter.
- New elements of control are added.
- There is more direct interaction with providers.
- Overhead cost and complexity increases in the health plan.

- There is greater control of utilization.
- Net rate of increase in medical costs is reduced.

While it would be comforting to classify all managed care into one of these categories, the American health care system has been mixing and matching these elements to a dizzying degree. Thus, the reader must recognize that managed care is malleable and take that into account as appropriate.

Types of Health Plans

Government Programs

In the United States in 1993, more than 40 percent of health care was provided or financed by federal and state governments. These programs include Medicare, Medicaid, military programs (direct care by military providers as well as the Civilian Health and Medical Program of the Uniformed Services [CHAMPUS]), the Federal Employee Health Benefits Program (FEHBP), the Veterans Administration, the U.S. Public Health Service, and some other programs. These programs may incorporate few to all managed care features, but they are not the topic of this chapter.

Self-Funded Plans

Insurance is a financial vehicle that protects the purchaser from unexpected costs, for which the insurer provides coverage at a premium rate that is calculated to cover those costs on average. Insurance, however, comes with a lot of other baggage. First, insurance is taxed by each state via a premium tax. Second, most states have passed mandated benefits laws that require insurance policies to provide coverage for defined diseases, providers, procedures, and so forth. Last, the cost of insurance is affected by the costs of everyone in the coverage "pool." In other words, if one group has high medical costs, the costs for all of the others goes up as well (the degree of that effect is determined by the type of policy, whether it is community-rated, experience-rated, and so forth).

The Employee Retirement Income Security Act (ERISA) allows large employers to assume the risk of medical costs themselves and thus not be subject to premium taxes or mandated benefits. Their cost is determined solely by the costs of their own group. It is most common for the large employer to contract with a third-party administrator (TPA) to perform the management activities. The TPA is often a large insurance company or Blue Cross Blue Shield plan, thus confusing both members and providers about who the insurer actually is. These large carriers provide not only administrative functions, but also substantial discounts to employers when the carrier has such discounts with providers. Self-funded plans may mimic any type of insurance coverage, as described below.

Traditional Insurance

Traditional insurance (which is rapidly becoming nontraditional) is basically of two types: indemnity insurance and service plans.

Indemnity Insurance

Indemnity insurance indemnifies the insured against financial losses from medical expenses. The only restriction is in the schedule of benefits. There are generally no restrictions on licensed providers. The insurance company reimburses the subscriber directly or may pay the provider directly, but it has no obligation other than to pay the subscriber. Professional reimbursement (i.e., payment to physicians and other professional providers) is subject to usual, customary, or reasonable (UCR) fee screens, while institutional reimbursement is generally based on charges.

Benefits are generally subject to deductibles (a flat dollar amount paid by the subscriber before any benefit is paid by the insurance company) and coinsurance (a percentage of the covered charge that is paid by the subscriber). Any charges that are not paid by the insurance company are strictly the responsibility of the subscriber.

Most indemnity plans require precertification of elective hospital admissions and may apply a financial penalty to the subscriber for failure to precertify. The plan may also perform some additional utilization management on hospital cases, but generally this is done over the telephone by plan-employed nurses located elsewhere. Large-case management may also be used to help control the cost of catastrophic cases. Mandatory second opinion programs may also be present for certain elective procedures (e.g., cardiac bypass surgery).

Costs for this type of health care coverage have been rising faster than those for any other type of health plan. As those costs rise, more people move into managed care.

Service Plan

The term "service plan" applies primarily, though not exclusively, to Blue Cross and Blue Shield Plans. In service plans, there are generally few restrictions on licensed providers who agree to sign a contract with the plan. The provider contract contains certain key elements: the plan agrees to reimburse the provider directly (eliminating collection problems with patients); the provider agrees to accept the plan's fee schedule as payment in full and not bill the subscriber for any payment not made by the plan (other than normal deductibles or coinsurance), and the provider agrees to allow the plan to audit the provider's records. Precertification, large-case management, and mandatory second opinion may be present and operate as they do for indemnity insurance.

The principal advantage of a service plan over indemnity insurance is the presence of provider contracts and reimbursement models that the contracts support. Professional fees are paid under a schedule of allowances that may, in effect, provide a discount to the plan. More important, the plan usually has significant discounts at hospitals that give it a competitive advantage. The hospitals grant these discounts for a variety of reasons, including large business volume; rapid payment; ease of collection; and, occasionally, advance deposits. Actual reimbursement to the hospital may be based on charges, per diems, diagnosis-related groups (DRGs), "cost plus," or some variation; these reimbursement methods are discussed later in this chapter.

Preferred Provider Organization

Preferred provider organizations (PPOs) are similar to service plans, with some important differences. The total panel of providers is reduced to some degree, often substantially. While the PPO may limit the number of providers in the network, there are two broad approaches: "any willing provider" versus criteria-based selection. In the former approach, any provider who wishes to participate and who agrees to the terms and conditions of the PPO's contract must be offered a contract, at least until the PPO feels it has adequate numbers of providers. In the latter approach, the PPO uses some objective criteria (e.g., credentials, practice pattern analysis, and so forth) that a provider must meet before a contract will be offered.

While reimbursement mechanisms to providers under PPOs may fall along the lines mentioned under service plans, in general the discounts are greater. It should be noted that many service plans require providers to give them "favored nation" pricing; in other words, a provider may not provide a better discount to a competitor than it does to the service plan. As a rule, PPOs do not place providers at risk for medical costs; the concept of risk-sharing with providers is discussed later in this chapter.

Precertification, large-case management, and mandatory second opinion are almost always present. The main difference is that failure to comply with these programs results in a financial penalty to the provider, not to the subscriber. As under service plans, a contracting provider may not bill the subscriber for any payment not made by the PPO, except for normal deductibles and coinsurance. In the event that a subscriber chooses to seek care from a nonparticipating provider, the responsibility then falls on the subscriber, who is at risk for any financial penalties and for charges not paid by the PPO.

A hallmark of PPOs is a benefits differential, commonly 20 percent, if a member sees a provider who is not in the PPO network. For example, if a member sees a network provider, coverage is provided at 90 percent of allowed charges; if a member sees a provider not in the network, the coverage may be at the 70 percent level.

There are two types of PPOs: risk-bearing and nonrisk-bearing. A risk-bearing PPO combines the insurance or payment function with management of the network of providers. A nonrisk-bearing PPO refers solely to the network and not to the insurance function. For example, a commercial insurer may build a network and sell coverage to clients; this would be an example of a risk-bearing PPO. Alternatively, a group of providers may come together as a legal entity; establish fee allowances, credentialing criteria, utilization review, and so forth; and contract with independent insurers to provide medical services to those insurers' customers; this would be an example of a nonrisk-bearing PPO.

Health Maintenance Organization

Health maintenance organizations (HMOs) are fundamentally different from the health plans described above. Although there are a few exceptions, known as "open-access" HMOs, that are similar in benefits design to PPOs, the vast majority of HMOs operate to further manage utilization and quality. It should be noted that HMOs often form the "in-network" portion of a point-of-service plan, which is described later. Benefits to members in an HMO are restricted (with some exceptions) to those provided by HMO providers and must be in compliance with HMO authorization procedures. Benefits obtained through the HMO tend to be significantly richer than those found in traditional insurance plans or in PPOs. Except for emergencies or unless specifically authorized, services received from non-HMO providers are the responsibility of the subscriber, not the HMO. Services rendered by contracting providers who fail to obtain proper authorization are the responsibility of the provider, who may not balance bill the member.

Traditional HMOs currently fall into two broad categories: open panel and closed panel. A third category, the network model, is common only in certain parts of the country, but it is likely to become more common in the future. Some HMOs mix model types in the same market. Open-access HMOs will be described briefly, and then traditional HMOs will be described in further detail.

Open-Access HMOs

Open-access HMOs are more like PPOs than traditional HMOs. In the open-access HMO model, members may access any provider in the HMO without going through a primary care physician (PCP). The PCP model is a hallmark of the traditional HMO. In the open-access model, members may see any PCP or specialist in the network on a self-referral basis. While this looks much like the PPO, in the open-access HMO, physicians share at least some level of risk for costs. Therefore, if professional costs exceed budget, physicians accept lower fees, lose their withholds, and so forth. It is theoretically possible to capitate specialists in this model, but it is extremely hard in practice because there is no reliable base to use for the capitation (in other words, members are not required to select specific PCPs or specialists, so actuaries cannot decide who should receive the capitation payment).

Open-access plans were popular in the late 1970s and early 1980s, especially with plans that were sponsored by organized medical societies. Unfortunately, these plans largely failed and suffered substantial losses because of high medical costs. There has been a recent revival of interest in open-access plans because of consumer demands. HMOs that are currently adopting these plan designs are doing so on the assumption that, because so few referral authorizations are denied, it is not worth the cost and may even raise the cost by adding an unnecessary PCP visit. This line of reasoning ignores the value in asking a PCP to make a judgment about the need for a referral rather than relying on a patient to make that judgment. In other words, it is assumed that all (or most) patient-generated requests for referral will be appropriate or will not be diverted by visiting a PCP. While open-access HMOs failed miserably in past years, it remains unknown if they will fare better now that physicians and hospitals are functioning more efficiently than in the past.

Open-Panel Plans

Open-panel HMOs contract with private physicians and other professional providers to see members in the providers' offices. The provider is an independent contractor and may contract with more than one competing health plan (and usually does), as well as have fee-for-service patients. The provider may be reimbursed through a variety of mechanisms. The total number of providers in an open-panel plan is larger than that of a closed-panel plan but usually smaller than in a PPO. Members must choose a single provider to be their PCP, sometimes referred to as a "gatekeeper," who must authorize any other services. A member may change PCPs at designated times if desired.

Open-panel plans fall into two broad categories: independent practice associations (IPAs) and direct contract models. While the terms are often used synonymously, they are technically distinct.

In an IPA, the HMO contracts with a legal entity known as an IPA, and pays the IPA a negotiated capitation amount. The IPA, in turn, contracts with private physicians. The IPA may reimburse the physicians through capitation or may use another mechanism, such as fee for service. Providers are at risk under this model, in that, if medical costs exceed the capitation amount, the IPA receives no additional funds from the HMO and must adjust reimbursement to providers.

In direct contract models, the HMO contracts directly with providers. The HMO reimburses the providers directly and performs all related management tasks. Direct contract models are currently the most common form of HMO.

Closed-Panel Plans

Closed-panel plans differ from open-panel plans in that the closed-panel plan uses physicians whose practices are confined to the HMO. These physicians practice from facilities that are likewise dedicated to the HMO. The total number of providers in the plan is by far the smallest of any model type. Members usually do not have to choose a single PCP but may see any PCP in the HMO (although they may be asked to choose a primary facility in order to provide continuity). Closed-panel plans fall into two broad categories: group model and staff model.

In group-model plans, the HMO contracts with a medical group to provide services to members. The HMO pays the group a negotiated capitation, and the group, in turn, reimburses physicians through a combination of salary and risk/reward incentives. The group is responsible for its own governance, and physicians are either partners in the group or associates. The group or the HMO provides the dedicated practice facilities and support staff, but most commonly it is the HMO's responsibility. The group is at risk in that, if the costs of the group exceed the capitation amount, reimbursement to providers is lowered, although the HMO generally provides stop-loss insurance coverage to protect the group from catastrophic cost overruns. Some groups exist primarily on paper and operate strictly as cost pass-through vehicles for the HMO, thus resembling staff-model plans.

In staff-model plans, providers are employees of the HMO. Physicians are reimbursed by salary, with an incentive plan of some sort. The HMO has full responsibility for management of all activities.

Network Model
The term network model is occasionally used to refer to an open-panel plan, but this section will discuss only the "true" network model, in which the HMO contracts with several large multispecialty medical groups for medical services. The groups are paid under capitation, and they, in turn, reimburse physicians under a plethora of mechanisms. The groups operate relatively independently. The HMO contracts with more than one group, but the number is usually limited.

Mixed Model
Many HMOs have adopted several model types, even in the same market, in order to capture additional market share. The most common form of mixed model involves grafting a direct-contract model to either a closed-panel or a network model. The HMO may also need to expand its medical service area and may choose to contract with private physicians rather than make the expenditures required for a facility. In mixed-model plans, the models often operate independently of each other.

Point-of-Service Plans
Point-of-service (POS) plans combine features of HMOs and traditional insurance plans. An archaic but still technically valid use of the term refers to a simple PPO arrangement, although the federal government appears to be the only entity that uses the term that way. In a POS plan, members may choose which system to use at the point they obtain services. For example, if the member uses his or her PCP and otherwise complies with the HMO authorization system, the benefits for services may be quite rich and require the member to pay only a minor copayment; if the member chooses to self-refer or otherwise not use the HMO system to receive services, the plan still provides insurance coverage but at a much lower level, such as requiring a deductible and coinsurance. The difference between in-network and out-of-network coverage for services generally ranges from 20 to 40 percent.

POS plans have been developed to resolve the conflicting issues of cost control and total freedom of choice of providers. By bringing the issue of cost differential directly to members at the point where they seek medical services, members become more active participants in the process. POS plans are discussed in detail in a separate chapter in this series.

Provider Reimbursement
The topic of reimbursement is varied and intricate. A common problem in managed care is that managers think up new and unique methods of reimbursement that theoretically will yield positive results, only to find that the health plan has no systems capability to support it. Even worse, the cost of programming to support the new reimbursement methodology may far outweigh any advantage it had in the first place.

A small section on this topic in a single chapter cannot possibly cover all of these variations in detail. A general overview will be presented, and the reader is urged to review other sources to obtain greater detail on this important topic. General topics regarding reimbursement, such as timeliness of payment, method of payment, and so forth, are assumed to be understood by the reader.

Hospital Reimbursement

As illustrated in table 1, below, a variety of methods of reimbursing hospitals in managed care is available. Figure 2, below, provides the relative distribution of the most popular methods of reimbursement. A very brief description of these methodologies follows.

Table 1. Models for Reimbursing Hospitals

- Charges
- Discounts
- Per diems
- Sliding scales for discounts and per diems
- Differential by day in hospital
- Diagnosis related groups (DRGs)
- Differential by service type
- Case rates or package pricing
  - Institutional only
  - Bundled
- Bed leasing
- Capitation or percent of revenue
- Penalties and withholds
- Outpatient care

Figure 2. Hospital Reimbursement in Managed Care

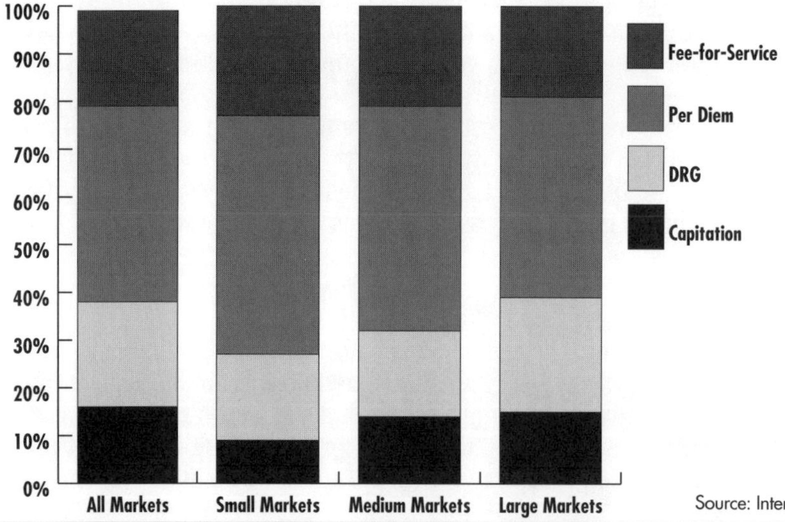

Source: Interstudy, 1995.

Straight Charges

The easiest method of payment is straight charges. It is also obviously the most expensive and the least desirable, after the option of no contract at all. In the past, some plans would agree to this simply to have a hospital in the network, but those days are fast fading.

Straight Discount on Charges

A common arrangement is a straight percentage discount on charges. In this case, the hospital submits its claim in full, and the plan discounts it by the agreed-to percentage. The hospital accepts the discounted amount payment in full and does not bill the member for the difference, except for allowed deductibles and coinsurance.

The presence of coinsurance in the discount setting has led to a serious dispute in a number of plans. The issue is, What does the coinsurance apply to: the full charges or the discounted amount? Unless the benefits contract clearly states that coinsurance is to be applied to full charges, regardless of what the plan ultimately pays, an argument can be made that the coinsurance should only apply to the discounted payment, since coinsurance is a percentage of the total payment.

Sliding Scale Discount on Charges

More common than straight discounts are sliding scale discounts. With a sliding scale, the percentage discount is reflective of total volume of admissions and outpatient procedures.

How the plan tracks the level of discount needs to be established. Some may wish to vary the discount on a month-to-month basis, but more common is quarterly, semiannually, or even yearly. One may track total bed days or number of admissions. Whatever is finally agree to, it must be a clearly defined and measurable objective.

Straight Per Diem Charges

Unlike straight charges, a negotiated per diem is a single charge for a day in the hospital, regardless of any actual charges or costs incurred. In this very common type of arrangement, the plan negotiates a per diem rate with the hospital and pays that rate without adjustments.

Hospital administrators are sometimes reluctant to add days in the intensive care unit or obstetrics to the arrangement unless there is sufficient volume of regular medical-surgical cases to make the ultimate cost predictable. In a small plan, or in one that is not limiting the number of participating hospitals, the hospital administrator is concerned that the hospital will be used for expensive cases at a low per diem, while competitors will be used for less costly cases. In such cases, one approach is to negotiate multiple sets of per diem charges based on service type (e.g., medical/surgical, obstetrics, intensive care unit, neonatal intensive care, rehabilitation, etc.) or a combination of per diem and flat case rate. Occasionally, a high-cost medical device becomes widely available after the per diem has been established; in such cases, it is possible to negotiate an outlier payment that equates to the cost to the hospital for the new device.

The key to making a negotiated per diem work is predictability. If the number and mix of cases can be accurately predicted, a per diem can be calculated accurately. The per diem is simply an estimate of the charges (or costs) for an average day in the hospital, minus the amount of discount the parties agree to.

Sliding Scale Per Diem

Like the sliding scale discount on charges discussed above, the sliding scale per diem is also based on total volume. In this case, an interim per diem is calculated. Depending on the total number of bed days in the year, the plan either pays a lump sum settlement at the end of the year or withholds an amount from the final payment to the hospital for the year to adjust for an additional reduction in the per diem from an increase in total bed days. Adjustments are made on a quarterly or semiannual basis to reduce any disparities caused by unexpected changes in utilization patterns.

Differential by Day in Hospital

Most hospitalizations are more expensive on the first day. For example, the first day for surgical cases includes operating suite costs, the operating surgical team costs (nurses, recovery, etc.), and so forth. This type of reimbursement method is generally combined with a per diem approach, but the first day is paid at a higher rate. This is not common, primarily because it is complicated, difficult to support on most claims systems, and should not be necessary if standard per diems have been calculated properly.

Diagnosis-Related Groups (DRGs)

As with Medicare, plans may use DRGs to pay for inpatient care. There are publications of DRG categories, criteria, outliers, and trim points (i.e., the cost or length of stay that causes the DRG payment to be supplemented or supplanted by another payment mechanism) to enable parties to negotiate a payment mechanism for DRGs based on Medicare rates or, in some cases, state-regulated rates. DRGs are perhaps better suited to plans with loose controls on utilization, because DRGs put the risk and reward solely on the hospital.

Service-Related Case Rates

Similar to DRGs, service-related case rates are a cruder cut. In this reimbursement mechanism, various service types are defined (e.g., medical, surgical, intensive care, neonatal intensive care, psychiatry, obstetrics, etc.) and the hospital receives a flat per-admission reimbursement for whatever type of service the patient is admitted to. If services are mixed, a prorated payment may be made (e.g., 50 percent of surgical and 50 percent of intensive care).

Case Rates or Package Pricing

Whatever mechanism is used for hospital reimbursement, a plan frequently finds it necessary to address certain categories of procedures and negotiate special rates.

The most common of these is obstetrics. It is common to negotiate a flat rate for a normal vaginal delivery, another rate for a cesarean section, and a blended rate for both.

Another area in which plans commonly wish to negotiate flat rates is specialty procedures at tertiary hospitals—for example, negotiating a flat rate for coronary artery bypass surgery or for heart transplants. These procedures, while relatively infrequent, are tremendously costly.

A broader but increasingly common and important variation is package pricing, which refers to an all-inclusive rate paid for both institutional and professional services. The plan negotiates a flat rate for a procedure (e.g., bypass surgery), and that rate is used to pay all parties that provide services connected with the procedure. Bundled case rates require a certain measure of cooperation and trust between a hospital and its medical staff, or at least some of the medical staff.

Bed Leasing

Bed leasing, a very uncommon reimbursement mechanism, refers to a plan's actually leasing beds from an institution, regardless of whether the beds are used or not. This ensures revenue flow to the hospital and access to at least some beds for the plan, and it is budgetable. It is perhaps best used in those situations where a plan is assured of a steady number of bed days, with little or no seasonality. The problem with bed leasing is that there is no real savings from reduced utilization, unless contract terms allow the plan to lease the beds back to the hospital if they are not being used.

Capitation or Percentage of Revenue

Capitation refers to reimbursing the hospital on a fixed per member per month (PMPM) basis to cover all institutional costs for a defined population of members. The payment may be varied by age and gender, but it does not fluctuate with premium revenue. Percentage of revenue refers to a fixed percentage of premium revenue (i.e., a percentage of the collected premium rate) being paid to the hospital, again to cover all institutional services. The difference between percentage of revenue and capitation is that percentage of revenue may vary with the premium rate charged and the actual revenue yield. In both cases, the hospital accepts the entire risk for institutional services for the defined membership base; if the hospital cannot provide the services itself, the cost for such care is deducted from the capitation payment.

In order for this type of arrangement to work, a hospital must know that it will serve a clearly defined segment of a plan's enrollment and that it can provide most or all of the necessary services to those members. In these cases, the primary care physician is clearly associated with just one hospital or with a group of linked hospitals.

Hospitals and physicians, through physician hospital organizations (PHOs) or other forms of IDSs, may come together to accept a full capitation contract with a managed care plan. While that may be attractive to a plan (assuming the PHO didn't actually form simply to be a union and thus drive costs up), the PHO must be careful to understand how the proceeds of the capitation will be distributed. It is common for the two parties in a PHO to feel that the other party deserves less capitation than they are receiving and for disputes to arise.

Point-of-service (POS) plans with an out-of-network benefit make capitation methods difficult to use, because capitation in a POS plan may mean having to pay twice for a service—once under capitation and again if the member seeks service outside of the network. In areas where there are no real alternatives to a certain hospital (e.g., a rural area or an area where a hospital enjoys a monopoly), this problem may not be material, but that is the exception. Capitation tied to percentage of admissions to the hospital may also attenuate this problem.

The other issue to be aware of in this arrangement is that some state insurance departments may consider full-risk capitation as excessive. It may be reasoned that, if the health plan is not actually assuming the risk for services, it isn't really the health plan at all, but only a marketing organization. In such a case, there may be a question as to who should hold the certificate of authority or license to operate the health plan.

Penalties and Withholds

As with physician services (see below), penalties or withholds are occasionally used in hospital reimbursement methods. Goals are set for average length of stay and average admission rate; Part of the payment to the hospital may be withheld, or, conversely, the plan may set aside a bonus pool. In any event, if goals are met or exceeded, the hospital receives its withhold or bonus, and vice versa. One complication with this arrangement is the possibility that a hospital can make its statistics look good by simply sending patients to other hospitals, similar to problems encountered with physician capitation. If a service area is clearly defined, or the hospital is capitated, it may be easier to apply a risk or reward program.

Outpatient Procedures

The shift from inpatient to outpatient care has not gone unnoticed by hospital administrators. As care has shifted, so have charges. In some cases, outpatient charges exceed inpatient charges. Most managed care plans will require this shift in charges to be negotiated so as not to lead to an unexpected increase in costs as utilization shifts to the outpatient arena. The most common reimbursement methods are discounts, flat charges, case rates, and capitation.

Professional Reimbursement

While there are fewer basic ways of reimbursing physicians and other professionals, there are countless variations on themes and numerous hybrids, not to mention some methods that will not even be described here. The problem of a health plan's being able to support new and unusual reimbursement methods is even more acute when dealing with professionals, because there are so many more of them. The three basic methods of paying physicians are salary, capitation, and fee-for-service.

Withholds, penalties, and incentive compensation may be applied to any of these methods.

Table 2, page 32, illustrates percentages of income from managed care for physicians who contract with different forms of managed care organizations. Figures 3 and 4, page 33, illustrate the predominance of the most popular of these forms of reimbursement at the time of this writing.

Salary

Salary is the predominant method in closed-panel plans, as well as in some group practices or situations in which physicians are employees (e.g., full-time faculty, government-employed physicians, or some full-time hospital-based physicians). Withholds may be applied to the base salary, and incentive plans are common.

Capitation

Although fee for service remains the most common form of reimbursement as this chapter is written, capitation continues to be a powerful and popular option for managed care. The use of capitation is generally confined to HMOs. Capitation is most easily applied to PCPs in HMOs (well over half of open-panel HMOs capitate PCPs), but it may be used for high-volume specialties as well.

Capitation payments are fixed payments made on a per member per month (PMPM) basis, regardless of the use of services. Payments are most often adjusted on the basis of age and gender of the member, because there is some correlation between those factors and utilization. Rarely, capitation may be adjusted on the basis of other factors, such as geographic location.

The key to capitation is the denominator: the number (and demographics) of the members for whom the provider is receiving capitation. That is why PCPs may be easily capitated in a model where the member must select a single PCP to provide and coordinate care. For specialists, there must be some mechanism to ensure that all of the members for whom capitation is being paid will not seek or receive services from a noncapitated provider (except under special circumstances).

Capitation paid directly to providers may be subject to a withhold, a portion of the payment held back by the plan to pay for any excessive utilization. Withholds are somewhat less common than they once were, as many managed care plan opt for programs based primarily on incentives rather than penalties.

Incentive payments are common in managed care plans, at least for PCPs. The incentive is most commonly tied to utilization, although incentives based on quality, access, and member satisfaction are being seen more often. The incentive is usually tied to a capitated pool of money that the plan applies against expenses in a defined category, such as referral or hospital costs. Money left in the pool at the end of the year is paid (in part or in whole) to physicians, either the entire panel of physicians or each individual physician, on the basis of utilization patterns. Variations on

Table 2. Managed Care Income for Providers Who Contract with MCOs

	Any [1]	HMO	IPA	PPO	Private Insurance[2]	Medicare	Medicaid
All	**33%**	**20%**	**11%**	**18%**	**44%**	**25%**	**5%**
Specialty							
Gen/FP[2]	35%	22%	17%	19%	45%	22%	6%
Gen/IM	32%	22%	11%	18%	40%	40%	5%
Gen Surg	32%	18%	11%	18%	45%	35%	5%
Pediatrics	44%	28%	13%	24%	50%	0%	17%
OB/GYN	44%	26%	12%	26%	62%	5%	5%
Radiology	26%	21%	11%	12%	40%	30%	8%
Psychiatry	37%	19%	11%	20%	33%	10%	2%
Anesthesiology	32%	20%	11%	14%	50%	25%	10%
Pathology	24%	18%	3%	15%	40%	30%	5%
EM	24%	19%	6%	9%	40%	25%	15%
Other	36%	19%	14%	18%	40%	20%	5%
Census Division							
New England	39%	23%	12%	12%	45%	30%	8%
Mid Atlantic	29%	22%	12%	12%	40%	25%	3%
East N. Central	28%	17%	11%	16%	42%	30%	5%
W. North Central	35%	22%	9%	22%	45%	30%	5%
S. Atlantic	30%	17%	9%	18%	40%	26%	5%
E. South Central	33%	13%	8%	23%	40%	30%	10%
W. South Central	33%	21%	5%	19%	44%	20%	5%
Mountain	41%	21%	11%	20%	50%	20%	5%
Pacific	41%	27%	15%	22%	50%	20%	5%
Practice Size							
1	31%	17%	11%	19%	40%	30%	5%
2-4	33%	18%	10%	19%	48%	30%	5%
5-9	33%	17%	13%	17%	50%	25%	5%
10-24	30%	19%	11%	15%			
25+	14%	36%	8%	14%			

1. *Physician Marketplace Statistics*, 1995 (1995 Socioeconomic Monitoring System core survey, nonfederal physicians). Chicago, Ill.: American Medical Association, 1996.

2. *AMA Socioeconomic Characteristics of Medical Practice*, 1996 (1995 Socioeconomic Monitoring System core survey). Chicago, Ill.: American Medical Association, 1996.

Figure 3. Compensation of Primary Care Physicians in Managed Care

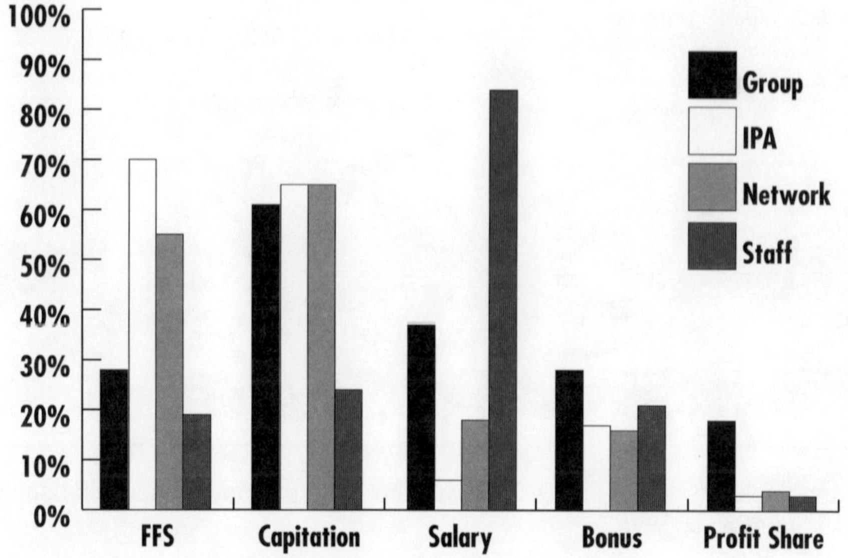

Source: Hoechst Marion Roussel, Inc. HMO-PPO Digest, 1995.

Figure 4. Compensation of Specialty Physicians in Managed Care

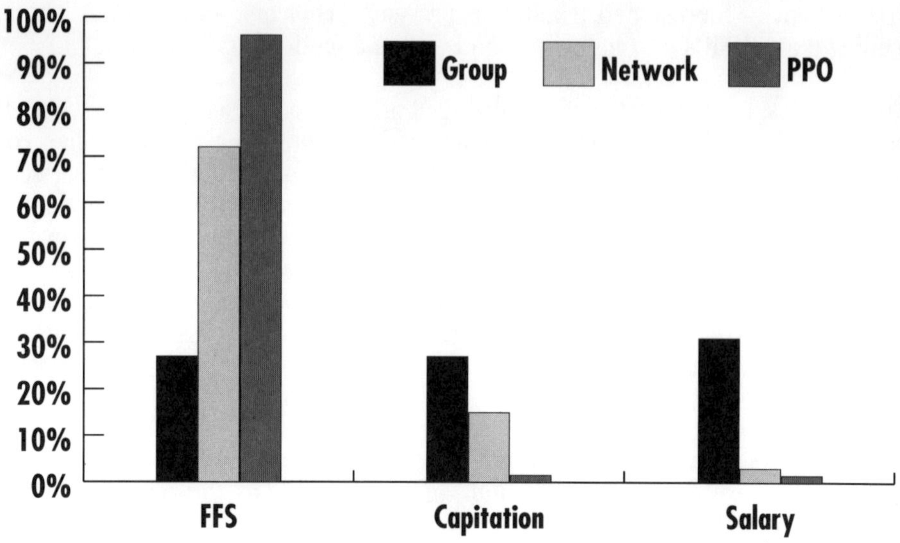

Source: Physician Payment Review Commission Mathematical Policy Research, Inc., and Medical College of Virginia, 1994

Figure 5. Capitation of Physicians in the United States

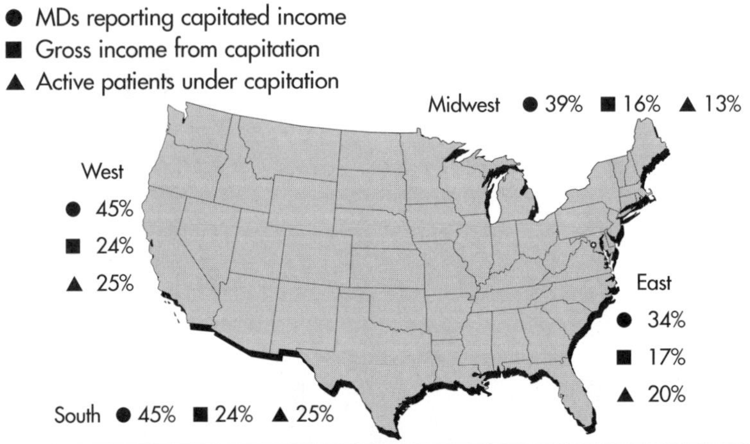

this approach are legion. Figure 5, above, illustrates the amount of capitation in the United States as of 1995.

Fee for Service

Fee for service remains a significant form of reimbursement in HMOs and nearly the only form of reimbursement in PPOs, service plans, and indemnity plans. While somewhat less than capitation in managed care, fee for service is not grossly antithetical to managed care. Even in HMOs that capitate PCPs, referral specialists are usually paid under fee-for-service arrangements. In managed care plans in which POS is heavily represented, capitation presents problems, as noted earlier, thus leading many HMOs to reimburse even PCPs on a fee-for-service basis.

Nevertheless, fee-for-service, if not managed properly or if used in a plan where the provider's first priority is to make money, can lead to increased costs when compared to capitation. Therefore, it is common for HMOs that use fee for service to place fees at some form of risk. A withhold on a percentage of the fee is the most common mechanism. If utilization exceeds budget, the withhold is used to cover the overage; if utilization is below budget, the withhold is paid out. Another form of risk is reductions in fees if utilization gets too high. Some plans have experimented with global fees (to avoid upcoding and unbundling) with some success. Other plans have tried adjusting a physician's fees on an individual basis according to that physician's utilization pattern.

Utilization Management or Care Management

Total health care costs may be thought of simplistically as the result of only two variables: price times volume. The preceding section briefly described issues germane to price; this section will briefly discuss volume—i.e., utilization. Management of utilization, sometimes referred to as care management, may be broadly divided into three categories: prospective, before the event occurs; concurrent, while the event is occurring; and retrospective, after the event has occurred.

Prospective Review

Prospective management of utilization applies to several major categories: health risk appraisals, demand management, referral services, and institutional services.

Health Risk Appraisals

Health risk appraisals (HRAs) are not new to most physicians, especially PCPs. HRAs have traditionally been used for an overall assessment of a new patient's medical condition and risk factors. In managed care, the same activity takes place, but the instruments are also designed to elicit information on member issues for which the plan needs to intervene in order to preserve health and lower overall costs. These appraisals may also be focused on specific lines of business, such as commercial members, Medicare members, and Medicaid members.

Many advanced Medicare HMOs go well beyond data-gathering forms and history and physical examinations and send a nurse or home health aide to the home of the new Medicare member. The nurse may do a nutritional assessment, check for compliance with prescribed medications, and so forth. The assessment may also look at simple interventions that can save problems later, such as providing an inexpensive bath mat to prevent the senior member from slipping in the tub and breaking a hip.

Demand Management

The most common methods of managing demand for medical services before such services are incurred include providing home care manuals, access to preventive services, and convenient hours of operation by providers. Recently, a more aggressive approach has shown considerable promise: provision of 24-hour-per-day nurse advice lines—access to a trained nurse on a 24-hour-per-day, 7-day-per-week basis through a toll-free number. Advice lines are often provided via contracts with companies that specialize in such services and rely heavily on clinical protocols. Many plans that use this service find that emergency department utilization is reduced.

Referral Services

Management of referral services is principally confined to HMOs, specifically to HMOs that use a PCP to coordinate care (the "gatekeeper" model discussed above). In this model, all care from any professional other than a PCP must be authorized by the member's PCP. The only physician the member may see without authorization is the PCP, although many plans make exceptions for obstetrics and gynecology and occasionally for mental health and substance abuse services. This authorization requirement allows the PCP to determine if the problem may be treated by the PCP. If a referral is required, the PCP utilizes a specialist under contract to the plan. The authorization is rarely open-ended, but rather for a limited number of visits (e.g., one to three) except in defined circumstances (e.g., chemotherapy may be fully authorized for all visits).

It is exceedingly rare for the plan to become involved in this process other than to capture the authorization data in order to process the claim properly. The PCP is expected to exercise proper clinical judgment without the plan's intervention. The plan should provide periodic reports to the PCP with data regarding referral rates and costs and information on the PCP's capitation pool or withhold if that is appropriate.

Institutional Services

Prospective management of institutional services, both inpatient and outpatient, is a staple of managed care in all types of plans. The procedure is simple. Someone calls the plan to request authorization for an elective admission or outpatient procedure; the plan checks it against clinical criteria and authorizes (or denies, although that is unusual) the procedure and a set amount of inpatient days as appropriate.

Who calls the plan depends on the type of plan. For indemnity plans or out-of-network benefits in PPOs and POS, the member must call or face an economic penalty. For HMOs and in-network benefits in PPOs and POS, the responsibility is on the provider, who must bear the economic penalty for failure to comply.

Clinical criteria for authorization are commercially available, or the plan may develop its own. Likewise, maximum allowable length of stay guidelines are commercially available, or the plan may modify guidelines to suit the local area. Most managed care plans are now using computerized programs to provide this information quickly and to capture pertinent data.

Concurrent Review

Concurrent review applies almost solely to inpatient care and large case management.

Inpatient Care and Continued Stay Review

Some plans, such as indemnity or service plans or PPOs, monitor active inpatient cases from a remote site via telephone. The plan's utilization management (UM) nurse will call the hospital to ascertain the status of the case. If the case is on track, no further action is taken. If the case is going to exceed the previously authorized days in the hospital, the UM nurse will collect clinical data and either authorize continued days or deny them. Many HMOs send UM nurses on-site to the hospital. This allows the nurse to obtain more detailed and timely information and to more actively help to manage the case.

In the event that there is any ambiguity or disagreement during this process, the UM nurse refers the case to a physician working with or for the health plan (either the medical director or a physician advisor). This physician may call the attending physician to discuss the case and may make a determination regarding authorization for further payments.

Large-Case Management
Some of the greatest cost savings potential in managed care is possible in large-case management, catastrophic or chronic cases that exceed routine costs by several orders of magnitude and in which active intervention by trained nurses at the plan can have a significant effect. Examples of such cases include acquired immune deficiency syndrome (AIDS), transplants, serious trauma, brittle diabetes, and so forth. The nurses at the plan are able to coordinate many aspects of care, such as rehabilitation, home care, health education, and the like, in order to better manage the case.

Disease Management
Disease management refers to a special form of large-case management. In this instance, the plan focuses on a handful of selected clinical conditions and works very proactively with the patient to control the course of the disease. This provides for greater continuity and better outcomes. Common examples of clinical conditions that receive attention include AIDS, insulin-dependent diabetes mellitus, childhood asthma, and congestive heart failure. The hallmark of these programs is the combined activities of numerous professionals, not just physicians. For example, a clinical pharmacist may be more active in childhood asthma than the pediatrician (e.g., teaching the child how to use inhaled steroids). Disease management differs from many preventive care activities in that the diagnosis is clear and cost savings occur concomitantly with improved outcomes (as opposed to, say cholesterol screening, where improved outcomes come at an enormous increase in cost).

Retrospective Review
Retrospective management refers to managing utilization after the utilization has actually occurred. It falls into two broad categories: case review and pattern analysis.

Case Review
Case review refers to review of individual cases for appropriateness of care, billing errors, or other problems. In some cases, a plan may place a provider on regular review if there is suspicion of regular improprieties.

Pattern Analysis
The plan may amass significant amounts of utilization data in order to determine if patterns exist. The patterns may be provider-specific, such as for over- or underutilization, or they may be planwide, such as an unanticipated increase in cardiac testing costs. After the pattern has been found, the reasons for it must be investigated so that action may be taken.

Managed care plans are now attempting to provide greater retrospective data to network providers to allow them to compare themselves to their peers and to modify their practices as appropriate. This form of feedback promises to be a powerful adjunct in helping to control health care costs.

Quality Management

Managed care plans vary by model type in their approach to medical quality management. Indemnity and service plans, and even PPOs, generally are somewhat less aggressive in managing quality than are HMOs, although, as with all generalizations, there are notable exceptions. As in utilization management, as model types progress through the continuum, greater attention is paid to the subject and more resources are expended in managing quality. Almost all plans begin the quality management process with credentialing of participating providers. In addition to credentialing, two general approaches to quality management exist, often in conjunction with each other: classic quality management and "new" approaches, such as total quality management or continuous quality improvement. This section will provide a very brief description of these approaches.

Credentialing

Credentialing refers to the activity of collating and reviewing the professional credentials of participating providers. For hospitals and institutions, this generally is confined to accepting accreditation of the Joint Commission for Accreditation of Health Care Organizations. For professionals, the plan does its own credentialing or may contract with a credentialing verification organization (CVO). In either case, it is common to collect data considered standard by the National Committee for Quality Assurance. Table 3, page 39, provides an example of data elements that an HMO may require. HMOs, like hospitals, also query the National Practitioner Data Bank.

Plans usually recredential every two years; basic data are reconfirmed, copies of current licenses and insurance face sheets are obtained, and changes are updated. Plans may also add data regarding member satisfaction, quality management, and administrative activities to the credentialing database.

Classic Quality Management

The classic approach to managing health care quality is based on the works of Avedis Donabedian of the University of Michigan. The three key elements of this approach are structure, process, and outcome.

Structure

Structure looks at the infrastructure of the plan as it relates to quality. Examples include the makeup of the medical record (e.g., presence of a drug allergies list, laboratory notes, and so forth), immunization records, access to care (e.g., how long it takes to get routine and urgent appointments), waiting times in the office, telephone responsiveness, and so forth. Structure studies are usually done through on-site review by the plan's quality management nurses. A special form of structure study relates to the effect of the utilization system on access to care—the plan performs studies to ensure that utilization is not inappropriately low and that the authorization system is not forming a barrier to necessary care.

Table 3. Basic Elements of Credentialing

- Training (copy of certificates)
  - Location of training
  - Type of training
- Specialty board eligibility or certification (copy of certificate)
- Current state medical license (copy of certificate)
  - Restrictions
  - History of loss of license in any state
- Drug Enforcement Agency (DEA) number (copy of certificate)
- Hospital privileges
  - Name of hospitals
  - Scope of practice privileges
- Malpractice insurance
  - Carrier name
  - Currency of coverage (copy of face sheet)
  - Scope of coverage (financial limits and procedures covered)
- Malpractice history
  - Pending claims
  - Successful claims against the physician, either judged or settled
- National Practitioner Data Bank status
- Medicare, Medicaid, and Federal Tax ID numbers
- Social Security number
- Locations and telephone numbers of all offices
- Hours of operation
- Yes/No questions regarding:
  - Limitations or suspensions of privileges
  - Suspension from government programs
  - Suspension or restriction of DEA license
  - Malpractice cancellation
  - Felony conviction
  - Drug or alcohol abuse
  - Chronic or debilitating illnesses
- Provisions for emergency care and back up
- Use of nonphysician (i.e., midlevel) practitioners
- In-office surgery capabilities
- In-office testing capabilities
- Areas of special medical interest
- Record of continuing medical education

Process

Process refers to how care is actually rendered. One common method is through medical care evaluations (MCEs), in which plan nurses review a sample of outpatient medical records in terms of practice parameters established by the quality management committee; these practice parameters are often specific to a particular disease or procedure. Degrees of compliance are measured and reported back to providers as well as to the plan. Similar reviews of inpatient care are also common.

Outcome

Outcome refers to the results of the care that is rendered. Plans generally look at outcome from two perspectives: planwide and adverse events. Adverse events refer to negative outcomes that could have been prevented, such as hospital-acquired infections. Planwide outcomes refer to whether or not the medical care is beneficial—for example, successful treatment of designated conditions in outpatient, good outcomes from hospitalized cases, and so forth. A special form of outcome is member satisfaction; the plan will regularly survey members, analyze complaints, determine overall satisfaction levels, and act on identified problems.

New Approaches to Quality Management

Managed care has adopted many of the tenets of the recent approach to industrial quality improvement, often referred to as total quality management or continuous quality improvement. These approaches lend themselves more to closed-panel plans than to open panels or PPOs when applied to clinical care, but all types of plans can benefit from these techniques as applied to business practices.

Other Operational Aspects of Managed Care

Managed care plans combine the operational activities of medical management with activities of an insurance company. To describe these activities would be to exceed the reader's patience with the material that may justifiably be found in a single chapter. Table 4, page 41, provides a listing of some of these, and table 5, page 41, provides a listing of common key management positions in a managed care plan.

The Numbers

Although the primary business of managed care is financing and delivering health care services, managed care plans cannot escape a reliance on numbers. Numbers are used to calculate premium rates, to track expenses, to track medical utilization, and generally to manage the business of the plan. The insurance industry, and the managed care industry in particular, use certain formats to track cost and utilization, in addition to the more common methods of net income, return on investment, and so forth.

Per Member Per Month

Per member per month (PMPM) is an exceedingly common unit of measurement. It refers to the number of "things" per applicable enrolled member (subscriber or dependent) per month. The "things" may be dollars or units of utilization, such as visits (although other measures of utilization are more common). Cost PMPM is the

Table 4. Other Operational Activities of a Managed Care Plan

- Claims
  - Efficiency
  - Throughput
  - Accuracy
  - Timeliness
  - Link to authorization system
  - Review process for pended claims
  - Explanation of benefits statements
- Management Information Systems (MIS)—computer and data support
  - Hardware
  - Software
  - Report generation
    - Medical utilization
    - Operational
    - Ad hoc versus routine
  - Support for reimbursement and utilization policies
- Membership and Billing
  - Enrollment and disenrollment processing
  - Eligibility checking
  - Evidence of coverage
  - Timely and accurate billing & reconciliations
- Finance
- Underwriting and pricing
- Marketing
- General administration
- Coordination of all activities
- Regulatory relations
- Member services
- Negotiations
- Strategic planning
- Office management
- Public relations

Table 5. Key Management Positions

- Chief Executive Officer, Executive Director, or Plan Manager
- Chief Financial Officer
- Medical Director
- Other management positions critical for success:
  - Claims manager
  - Customer services manager
  - Utilization management manager
  - Quality management manager
  - Data and systems manager
  - Provider relations manager
- Other management positions required depending on plan configuration
  - Marketing director
  - Legal support
  - Facilities manager
  - Manager of medical support staff

most common use of the format. For example, if the plan has 50,000 members and is spending $600,000 per month on primary care services, the cost is $12 PMPM

While cost is generally applied over all enrolled members, plans may restrict the measurement to members to whom the measure applies. As an example, general medical costs for primary care services would apply to all members in the plan, while pharmacy services may only apply to 75 percent of enrolled members. In that case, the plan would report PMPM pharmacy costs using only those members who had the benefits; otherwise a misleadingly low PMPM cost would be reported.

Per Member Per Year

Similar in concept to PMPM, this measure is used not only for dollar costs, but for measuring utilization as well. For example, pharmacy costs may be reported as averaging 5.2 prescriptions PMPY, at a cost of $9.04 PMPM; simple arithmetic also yields two other common measures: $108.48 PMPY and $20.86 per prescription (this plan needs a pharmacy director!).

Per Thousand Members Per Year

This unit of measurement applies almost solely to utilization. It is used to track units of utilization on an annualized basis. The most common example is bed days per thousand members per year, usually referred to simply as bed days per thousand (and often abbreviated as BD/K). This is the total number of inpatient days used by an average one thousand members in a year. A typical HMO might report 300 bed days per thousand, meaning that for every one thousand members in the HMO, 300 inpatient days will be incurred. Because most plans calculate this number every month, a formula must be applied to annualize one month's data, both for a single month and average per month for the year to date.

Related to bed days per thousand are admissions per thousand. For example, a typical HMO might incur 78 admissions per thousand. If the plan reports 300 bed days per thousand, the average length of stay is 3.8 days. Other examples of this format include outpatient visits per thousand, surgical procedures per thousand, and so forth.

Other Measurements

Financial measurements track not only utilization costs and direct costs, such as the cost of administration, but also costs for which no complete record yet exists. A risk-bearing plan must accrue a liability each month for medical costs, even when claims have not yet been submitted. These costs are referred to as Incurred But Not Reported (IBNR) costs. If a plan fails to accrue such expenses, it will seriously underestimate the true cost of health care and not have enough money to pay claims.

Premium Rate Development and Budgeting

Premium rate development and budgeting is a requirement of any risk-bearing health plan. Using combinations of historical trends, actual prior experience, and management estimates of future costs, the plan must create premium rates to apply to its products. A wide variety of mechanisms exists to calculate different types of rates (e.g., community rates, adjusted community rates, rate banding, experience rates, minimum premium rates, administrative services only rates, and so forth).

Practical Suggestions and Strategies

There are many practical strategies and options that an individual health care provider should pursue in order to succeed in managed care. The following issues are worth discussing here.

Consolidation

Continued consolidation is occurring in the health care industry today. As physicians come out of training, they are often saddled with financial obligations that make it difficult if not impossible to go into solo practice or even to join small groups. Therefore, it is important for physicians to understand the value of joining with others. The negotiating advantages of large groups are obvious (though certainly not guaranteed by any measure!), but there are additional reasons and advantages.

Economies of scale can be achieved by larger groups. This is not always the case, and in fact many groups end up spending more overhead on administration rather than less, but the additional value of professional management is significant. The ability of a large group or organization of physicians to collect and use data and information is likewise enhanced.

Groups or large organizations also have greater ability to observe and manage the behavior of physician members. This may be seen as threatening by some physicians, but change must and does occur, and change driven by peers is preferable to change imposed from without.

Risk Assumption

Migration from fee-for-service reimbursement to capitation or other forms of performance-based reimbursement means changing the focus from episodic to continuous and from cost-based to resource-conserving. In order to benefit economically from the margin that is built in to most risk forms of reimbursement, physicians need to change how they view patients.

Physicians who accept risk for medical care must understand that, while a patient in this arena is always a member, a member is not necessarily a patient. This has a profound impact on how one provides service. It is most common for physicians to accommodate their sickest patients when they ask for service. For instance, if a chronically ill patient calls for an appointment, he or she is likely to get one relatively soon. This is as it should be; a physician's first responsibility is to care for the sick.

But what about the healthy? Most busy physician offices are not nearly as accommodating. If a new member under a capitated HMO calls for a first visit physical, or perhaps calls with minor symptoms, the most likely response will be to tell that person that they cannot get in, or cannot get an appointment for months. The new member is left unsatisfied.

The problems with this should be obvious. In any risk-sharing-reimbursement, capitation, or performance-based program, it is premiums paid by the healthy that pay for care of the sick. If healthier members do not feel that they are receiving value, they are very likely to change physicians, or even change health plans, thus depriving the pan of needed premiums.

Patients may be loyal to a physician, but there is a relationship between how sick a patient is to how loyal they will be. Members who rarely visit a physician have no loyalty at all, because they have other needs to address (for example, buying food, paying for a car, funding a child's education, and so forth) and are most likely to change health plans. When that happens, physicians are left with the sickest members, otherwise known as adverse selection.

Resource Management

Physicians must change their thinking to overall management of medical resources rather than just costs or charges. This is something that has been occurring for several years anyway, but it is heightened under managed care. And what occurs in the office is often only a minor part of the total use of medical resources. More important is what occurs in the broader picture of medical care: diagnostic testing, invasive procedures, specialty use, facility use, pharmaceuticals, etc. Most advanced managed care organizations realize this and are far more concerned with total medical resource use over episodes of care for good outcomes. Physicians need to think likewise.

Attitude

Is managed care a threat or a menace? Physicians who still have that attitude will hate their practice environment and will not thrive economically. Physicians must understand that in large measure, the changes that are required in practice behavior are more in habits than in science or even judgment. While always keeping the well-being of the patient foremost, physicians must be willing and able to recognize when they are resisting changing practice behavior because of habit or convenience.

Conclusion

Managed care and the U.S. health care system are in a rapidly evolving state. It is possible, however, through intelligent application of management, to provide good access and high quality at an acceptable cost. This is the goal of managed health care.

Bibliography

Boland, P., Editor. *The Capitation Sourcebook*. Berkeley, Calif.: Boland Healthcare, Inc., 1996.

Couch, J. *Health Care Quality Management for the 21st Century*. Tampa, Fla.: American College of Physician Executives, 1991.

Donabedian, A. *Explorations in Quality Assessment and Monitoring*. Chicago, Ill.: Health Administration Press, 1982.

Doyle, R. *Healthcare Management Guidelines.* Seattle, Wash.: Milliman & Robertson, Inc., 1990.

Eisenberg, J. *Doctor's Decisions and the Cost of Medical Care.* Chicago, Ill.: Health Administration Press, 1986.

Goldfield, N., and others. *Measuring and Managing Health Care Quality: Procedures, Techniques, and Protocols.* Gaithersburg, Md.: Aspen Publishers, 1991.

Kongstvedt, P., *The Managed Health Care Handbook, Third Edition.* Gaithersburg, Md.: Aspen Publishers, 1996.

Nash, D. *The Physician's Guide to Managed Care.* Gaithersburg, Md.: Aspen Publishers, 1994.

Pauly, M., and others. *Paying Physicians: Options for Controlling Cost, Volume, and Intensity of Services.* Chicago, Ill.: Health Administration Press, 1992.

Peter R. Kongstvedt, MD, FACP, is Partner, Ernst and Young, LLP, Washington, D.C.

Chapter 3

Health Maintenance Organizations

by Diana Barrett, DBA

Background

Although the dramatic realignment of relationships among providers, payers, and consumers termed "managed care" encompasses a broad range of incentives and organizational structures,[1] the fundamental objective of managed care is to restructure the way in which health services are organized in order to decrease costs, maintain quality, and provide access to the patient. Considerable controversy exists about all of these issues, from the definition of managed care itself to the degree to which the patient actually benefits from this reorganized care and, finally to the issue of cost savings. In this chapter, we will trace the development of a type of managed care arrangement known as the health maintenance organization (HMO). We will begin by tracing its history and development and then examine its success from various vantage points—that of actual and potential patients, sometimes referred to as "society," and that of health care providers who are or might be a part of an HMO. Finally, we will close with some conclusions about what role these organizations might play in the future.

Origins

The organization referred to as an HMO originated with the development, both in the United States and abroad, of prepaid health plans. The Kaiser health care system and Group Health Cooperative of Puget Sound in Seattle, founded by consumers, exemplify early efforts at organizing health care systems that avoided the traditional fee-for-service incentive structure and that focused on organizing patient use of services. Because the HMO is so often associated with Kaiser, it might be useful to trace the role that Henry Kaiser played in initiating this form of health care delivery.

Kaiser was a key pioneer, a major American industrialist who, in 1930, was expanding in both the steel and cement industries in California. In order to provide health care for a rapidly growing work force, he contracted with groups of full-time physicians to provide comprehensive care for his employees, going so far as to build hospitals and clinics. Physicians worked on salary, with bonuses based on their productivity. Consequently, the venture could be budgeted, planned, and staffed like any other business activity. During World War II, Kaiser's steel, cement, and shipbuilding ventures grew significantly, and so did his innovative health care system.

After the war, as his work force began to shrink from its wartime high, the Kaiser health care system, which expanded in Hawaii as well as on the West Coast, had excess capacity. Consequently, the Kaiser-Permanente Health Care System was "spun off" as an independent nonprofit corporation and soon began to provide health care for other companies.[2]

The Kaiser system was, of course, not unique. The Health Insurance Plan of New York was similar, and the Mayo Clinic, in Rochester, Minnesota, was a multispecialty group of salaried doctors.[2] The key difference is that none of these plans offered total coverage to a defined population for a fixed fee, a concept that we now refer to as capitation. In fact, the term HMO is a rather broad term and encompasses a number of arrangements by which an independent provider organization contracts with an employer to provide care (see table below). Various forms of HMOs have developed, but the initial concept has not changed: costs are controlled by providing incentives to do less rather than more, and care is delivered in a structure that stresses control via a "gatekeeper." This person's job is to control the use of expensive tests and, in theory, to maintain the health of the patient by screening and prevention in order to avoid future high costs of caring for untreated disease.

Nationwide Enrollment in Four HMO Model Types

	1993		1992		1991	
	Plans	Enrollment (000)	Plans	Enrollment (000)	Plans	Enrollment (000)
Group	68	14,011.9	71	11,368.2	73	11,190.3
IPA	351	24,021.7	363	21,183.9	365	18,171.1
Network	68	6,116.8	72	6,909.4	84	6,419.9
Staff	53	4,837.8	56	4,911.1	59	4,606.9
Total Operating	540		562		581	
Developing	2		2		4	
Total U.S.	**542**	**48,987.1**	**564**	**44,372.6**	**585**	**40,388.3**

Source: SMG Marketing Group, Inc., 1994
Enrollment figures are rounded and are based on the Marion Merrell Dow *Managed Care Digest, Update Edition,* 1993.

In the prepaid group practice model, the health benefits intermediary, such as the Kaiser Foundation Health Plan, Inc., has an exclusive relationship with one or more large groups, whereas, in a network model, such as Pacificare Health Systems, the relationship is nonexclusive. In a staff-model HMO, such as the Group Health Cooperative, the health benefit intermediary directly employs health care providers. In an independent practice association (IPA) HMO, such as Aetna U.S. Healthcare, Inc., the intermediary contracts with solo or small group practitioners. In a mixed-model HMO, such as Prudential Health Care Plans, the intermediary has various relationships with providers, some exclusive and others less so. Regardless of the organizational arrangement, prepaid systems were meant to incorporate financing mechanisms and the resources necessary to provide care to an enrolled population. From the beginning, managing care to this extent has involved far more than a change in financial incentives. Ultimately, it represents a restructuring of the health care system itself.

In the United States, early prepayment programs focused on a closed panel, a form of prepayment that was viewed as quite antithetical to traditional principles of capitalism. Consequently, health care providers employed in prepaid settings were often viewed with suspicion by their colleagues. Consumers have traditionally not been enthusiastic about joining these staff-model plans, which require use of specific physicians in a specific location, with inpatient care provided at one or more designated hospitals. In fact HMO enrollment figures show that, before 1980, fewer than 10 million Americans belonged to HMOs. By the end of 1994, an estimated 55 million Americans were HMO members (figures 1 and 2, page 50). Perhaps in response to this unwillingness to join closed-panel HMOs, the growth of point of service plans (POS), hybrid HMOs that permit members to use doctors outside of a network in return for paying a higher fee, has been particularly impressive.

While enrollment in HMOs and POS plans continues to rise, the prospects for the long-term success of the nation's roughly 600 preferred provider organizations (PPOs) is uncertain. One major reason is that PPOs are structured on a discounted fee-for-service basis. Doctors are paid on the basis of the services they deliver and therefore have no incentive to limit either patient visits or the number of procedures performed. Usually, there is no gatekeeper to coordinate care, control access to specialists, or eliminate duplication of diagnostic tests. Consequently, PPOs have a more difficult time holding down costs and ensuring that patients receive only care that is appropriate and necessary.[3]

While Kaiser initiated the concept of prepaid, all-inclusive care, the term HMO was coined by Paul Ellwood, a pediatric neurologist, and formally established through federal legislation during the administration of President Richard M. Nixon. As with wage and price controls that were being utilized at the time to reduce the inflation rate in the general economy, the establishment of HMOs was seen as an attempt to reduce health cost increases and to control utilization of services. Corresponding state legislation required employers to offer employees an HMO option if certain criteria were met. The HMO Act of 1973 required employers of 25 or more workers to

Figure 1. Health Maintenance Organization Growth

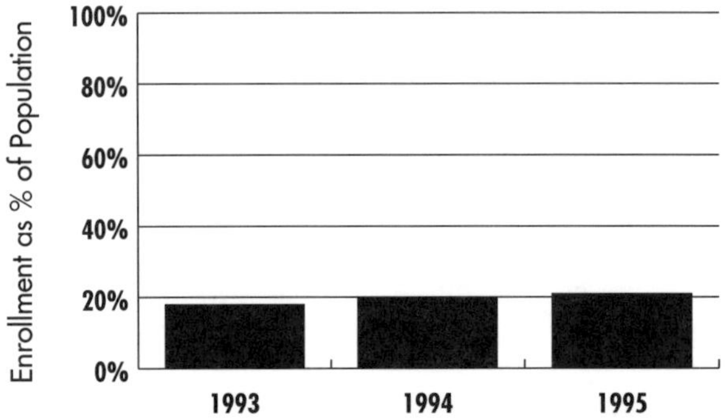

Source: 1993 data: GHAA, *National Directory of HMOs*, June 1994. 1994 and 1995 data: *Business & Health*, January 1995, Vol. 13, No. Speiss, Page 24, *The State of Health Care in America*, 1995.

Figure 2. HMO Enrollment Trends

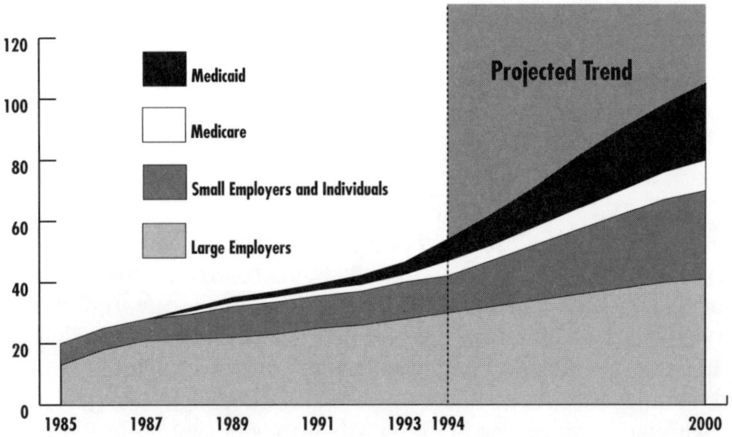

Source: *HMOs 1995: The Right Place, the Right Time, the Right Idea*, Robertson Stephens and Co., San Francisco, 1994

offer one group practice HMO and one individual practice HMO, if such organizations served their areas and asked to be offered. Ironically, many employers today offer only managed care options to their employees.

HMO Performance

There is little doubt about the prevalence of managed care (figure 3, page 51). In Massachusetts, for example, 39 percent of the population is enrolled in HMOs, and five other states show enrollment of more than 30 percent. Considerable questions exist, however, as to the performance of different managed care models.

- Do they in fact reduce costs?
- Is care made more readily accessible to a broader group of patients?
- Is quality improved?
- Do HMOs select healthier patients to begin with than do fee-for-service plans?

A number of studies have been done in an attempt to answer these questions. The RAND Health Insurance Experiment (RHIE)[4] as well as a number of later studies have examined managed care plan performance.[5] In general, researchers have tended to test the hypothesis that HMO plans have lower utilization and expenditures relative to indemnity plans. Because of the potential negative impact of decreased resource use on quality of care, researchers have also tested the hypothesis that HMO plans produce less favorable quality of care than do indemnity plans.[5] The results of those studies indicate that HMO plans have generally had somewhat lower hospital admission rates than indemnity plans, shorter lengths of stay, lower hospital days per enrollees, and lower use of expensive procedures. Findings in these areas were mixed, however, and even more so in the area of physician office visits per enrollee. While many studies have been done, some are based on a small number of observations, which limits their usefulness. Other studies have shown

Figure 3. Penetration of HMOs in the United States

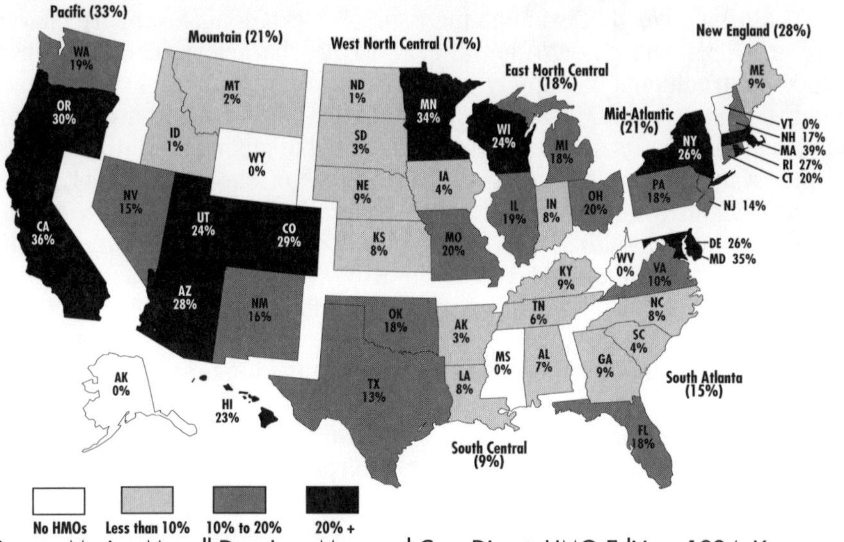

Source: Marion Merrell Dow Inc., Managed Care Digest, HMO Edition, 1994, Kansas City, MO, and SMG Marketing Group Inc., Chicago.

conflicting results. Data are similarly scarce on the impact of HMOs on national or regional area health care expenditures, with some studies showing no statistically significant relationship to hospital expenses per capita or per admission and others concluding that an increase in HMO market penetration led to a smaller increase in hospital costs per admission. In other words, this study suggested that HMO plans produced their effect on national or regional health care expenditures by reducing the growth rate of indemnity plan hospital expenditures.

One of the touted benefits of HMO plans has been their ability to provide preventive services.[6] A number of studies have shown that this indeed seems to be the case: HMO plan enrollees appear to receive more preventive tests, procedures, and examinations, as well as health promotion activities, such as smoking cessation counseling, than do indemnity plan enrollees.[7] As for quality of care, an area that is of perhaps the greatest interest to health care providers, both the question and the answer are complex. Assuming that the data describe the same outcomes or processes of care, there is evidence that HMOs and indemnity plans provide enrollees with roughly comparable quality of care. As for enrollee satisfaction, data suggest that fewer HMO enrollees than fee-for-service enrollees were satisfied with their perceived quality of care. After examining a broad array of studies, Miller and Luft conclude that HMO plans exhibit lower utilization of hospital services and of more expensive and discretionary tests, increased use of preventive services, and somewhat mixed results on health outcomes.[5]

The issue of adverse selection has, similarly, received a great deal of attention. Are persons who consume relatively few health services more or less likely to enroll in an HMO? Most studies that examine the issue of selection bias compare characteristics of enrollees who chose to enroll in HMOs to characteristics of persons who remained in traditional indemnity plans. Given the number of plans that are attempting to attract the Medicare population, it would be useful to better understand the characteristics of older persons interested in joining an HMO compared to those that want no part of managed care. Studies of enrollees in four Medicare Capitation Demonstrations—Group Health Cooperative of Puget Sound, Washington; Fallon Community Health Plan, Massachusetts; Kaiser Permanente, Portland, Oregon; and Greater Marshfield, Wisconsin—revealed that enrollees usually experienced lower rates of utilization during the period immediately preceding enrollment. A later study found that the relative risk of mortality was significantly lower for persons in those plans than for those who remained in the fee-for-service system.[8]

The underlying mechanism here may be relatively simple; healthy elderly people are far more likely than their unhealthy counterparts to consider joining an HMO, but, a few years down the line, the advantage of this self-selection process will disappear, given the likely need for medical services as both populations age. In terms of the nonelderly population, self-selection again seems to play a large role. Patients covered by an indemnity plan are more likely to have a chronic illness than are patients covered by an HMO. In one study, patients choosing an HMO option were found to have incurred reimbursement amounts, for the year prior to the choice, 54 percent lower than employees who remained with the traditional indemnity plan. Perhaps healthier people might be attracted to plans that emphasize health prevention and health maintenance. In fact, HMOs do offer more comprehensive benefits, primarily for routine checkups and minor illnesses. For persons who are not ill, these factors are likely to be important and to serve as a way of distinguishing among options—proxies for quality in the absence of other data. It must be remembered that, for many consumers, choices have been severely limited. The number of employers who still offer fee-for-service plans is small, and, even among managed care options, an increasing gap in premium costs among plans has minimized real choice, if one assumes that choice is largely a function of costs.

Given the potential of HMOs to control costs, private employers have embraced managed care as their preferred approach to moderating the growth of health insurance premiums (figure 4, below). In fact, the willingness of employers to embrace this change with such enthusiasm would suggest that there should be a significant reduction in the increase in national health care spending. This has not happened, so other forces are clearly at work. In contrast to the idea that consumers have increasingly limited choice, Enthoven, for example, argues that consumers have lacked sufficient incentive to choose an HMO. He believes that factors such as employer coverage practices, the existing tax code, and the number of coverage options per purchasing group have reduced purchaser's sensitivity to price and thereby decreased the plans' incentives to cut costs.[9] In other words, he believes that consumers have not had a clear financial reason to choose an HMO and employers have lacked sufficient incentive to price their choices in such a way that HMO rather than indemnity might be the preferred choice. The terrain has changed so dramatically, however, that insufficient choice for consumers is today becoming the common reality. Organizations that once offered a range of plans, including at least one fee-for-service plan, today might offer a small number of managed care options with one high-priced indemnity plan that has a strong "managed care" component as well.

Figure 4. Decline in HMO Premiums

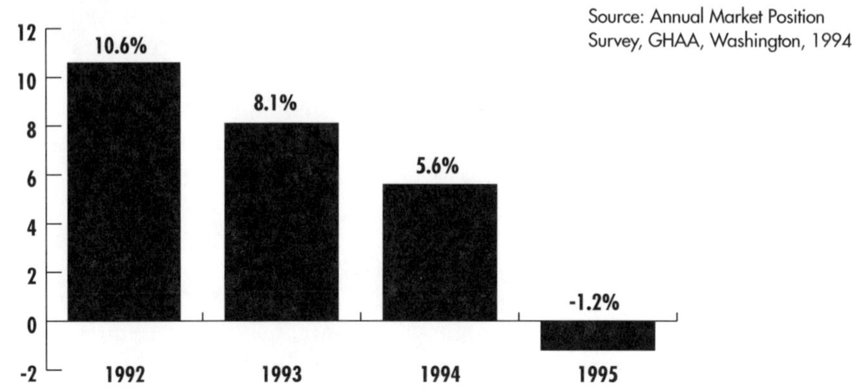

Typically, employers offered HMOs and paid their premiums in full, as long as the premiums did not exceed those of traditional coverage. Either way, coverage was essentially free to employees. The incentive in this situation was for the HMO to "shadow price"—an interesting concept that can be defined as the decision to set a price just below the price of another service that is likely to be purchased, in this case that of indemnity coverage. Particularly efficient HMOs, or those that paid special attention to quality or to preventive services, were no more likely to be offered, or chosen, than plans that were merely less expensive. Employers and employees view the choice of coverage as a financial and an insurance problem, not as a choice among different organizations of care. In fact, because the comparative costs for the consumer of two different plans do not necessarily reflect quality or service differences between those plans, choice has generally been made on the basis of meager information, generally the cost of the premium.

Traditionally, little information has been available about such issues as continuity of care (the same physician available over time), quality of care based on measurable outcomes, patient satisfaction studies, or actual differences among plans. The existing federal tax code exacerbates this problem. Premium contributions are "employer-paid" contributions made in before-tax dollars, providing little incentive for employees to choose HMO rather than indemnity coverage. They have similarly reduced the incentive for HMOs to differentiate themselves in the marketplace on the basis of real quality differences, particularly when these quality differences might go unnoticed in a population that often changes health plans with each change of employer. In fact, true differentiation on the part of an HMO, such as advertising suggesting a particular strength in care of diabetes or joint disease, could in fact lead to a disproportionately high number of patients with medical conditions that are costly to treat.

Yet, evidence does appear to exist suggesting that, if all acute health care services were delivered through staff- or group-model HMOs, national health spending might be almost 10 percent lower.[10] Of course, this says nothing about the quality of services in an HMO setting. Looking at the care of chronically ill children, for example, the data are complex and often conflicting. In one study that addressed how well HMOs met the needs of almost 700,000 children with disabilities due to chronic conditions,[11] HMOs offered better protection than conventional plans against out-of-pocket expenses and were much more likely than fee-for-service plans to cover ancillary therapies, home care, outpatient mental health care, and medical case management. In addition, few HMOs maintained exclusions for preexisting conditions.

Other aspects of HMO policies, however, were found to operate against the interests of families with chronically ill children. HMOs commonly made specialty services available only when significant improvement was expected within a short period. Also, limits were placed on the availability of mental health and other services frequently needed. Perhaps the most difficult problem for these children and for their families was the lack of choice among and access to appropriate specialty providers.

It appears that availability and quality of services available to a child with special needs is likely to depend on the parent's ability to maneuver within the system.

Similar questions can be asked about mental health services in HMOs.[12] Rapid changes and proliferation of managed care plans has created a bewildering climate for psychotherapists and for psychiatry in general. Fearful of being excluded from managed care plans, many therapists have fallen silent, agreeing to practices they do not support. Psychiatrists have had to depend on a combination of pharmacology and an abbreviated course of therapy, combined with extremely limited inpatient care to treat an increasingly complex population.

The Patient's Perspective

From the patient's point of view, choice of physician is of greatest interest. Consumers will be reluctant to alter their coverage if it means that they can no longer see their chosen physician, regardless of the quality of care they are receiving from this provider or that, in any given year, approximately 25 percent of Americans change residences, often requiring a change in primary care provider. In fact, the higher percentage of younger families in managed care plans may reflect that they are less likely to have an established relationship with a physician. This fact, coupled with lower out-of-pocket costs and a greater interest in comprehensive benefits, will lead to higher enrollment in HMOs.

In a recent study conducted by the Commonwealth Fund,[13] the authors found that minorities were also more likely to be enrolled in managed care plans. Fee-for-service and managed care respondents reported similar health status, although fee-for-service enrollees were older. More families choosing managed care reported cost to be an important factor in their decisions, while perceived quality of physicians was important factors for both fee-for-service and managed care insured families. The survey revealed high rates of plan changing, mostly because of changes in employment. This survey found no significant differences in terms of satisfaction with care. Past comparative studies have generally found lower levels of satisfaction and perceived quality of care for managed care enrollees than for their counterparts in fee-for-service plans. However, most of these studies have used the Medicare or Medicaid population or a single large employee group rather than a population across different employment groups.

In the above survey, respondents appeared to be reasonably satisfied with their health insurance, whether in managed care or fee-for-service plans. However, managed care enrollees reported lower overall ratings than those in fee-for-service plans, rating both their plan, quality received, and access to care less highly than did fee-for-service enrollees. Aggregated numbers, however, often do not tell the whole story, however. A range of factors make up a patient's perception of quality, including satisfaction with care for a serious illness, satisfaction with an individual physician, time spent with a provider, the ability of providers to listen, and phone accessibility. On all of these measures, enrollees rated fee-for-service plans more highly than managed care plans.

In another study involving five practice types,[14] patients in solo fee-for-service practices rated their outpatient visits best and HMO patients rated theirs worst. Whether fee-for-service or prepaid, care was rated better in small than in large practices. These responses were directly related to disenrollment and in fact could be used to predict which patients, when given the option, would choose to disenroll.

How well do patients understand their health care coverage in the first place? Data from two surveys[15] suggest that almost all privately insured persons understand the basic elements of their insurance plans but underestimate their coverage for mental health, substance abuse, and prescription drug benefits and overestimate their coverage for long-term care. People who are newly enrolled in HMOs seem uncertain about what services their plans cover and restrictions on their choice of hospitals.

The Health Care Provider's and Hospital's Perspective

Issues of provider performance and patient satisfaction are complex, yet a discussion of the HMO as a major player in the managed care scenario would be incomplete without discussing the role of health care providers in this structure.

- How do clinicians working in HMOs view their degree of clinical freedom, satisfaction with income, status in their profession, autonomy, resources, and professional relations?
- Are they satisfied, and does this level of satisfaction appear to vary by specialty?

In one study,[16] 850 physicians were interviewed and their level of satisfaction appeared high, with little difference noted among specialties. The only difference appeared to be in satisfaction with income, with primary care specialists predictably less satisfied than surgical specialists. It should be noted that this study was done in Dane County, Wisconsin, an area that has experienced a decline in independent practice, limiting choice for physicians.

Physicians seem to fall into three general groups in terms of their relationship with managed care. The groups are a function of the competitive characteristics of the area in which they live and work as well as their personal needs, training, and aspirations. The first group remains philosophically opposed to the basic principles of managed care and will continue to make every effort to remain in private practice—a feat that is certainly easier in some geographical areas than others. The second group is generally skeptical about the touted benefits of managed care and would like nothing better than to keep its distance, but it also realizes than, in its market area, this route is becoming increasingly problematic. The third group is made up of physicians who have established for themselves and for the group of professionals important to them that managed care, including HMOs, is a permanent fixture in the landscape of American medical practice. They are optimistic about their role in this restructured arena and want to maximize the level of control they have.

It should also be noted that age, training, and probably gender play a role in the degree to which physicians are or are not willing to participate in this arena. A recent study of more than 600 first-year medical students in California found considerable acceptance of health care reform. They felt that practicing physicians had a major responsibility to help reduce costs. They were particularly enthusiastic about reform of the malpractice system and about increased spending on preventive health services as the steps most likely to be effective. Although only a small number of the students wanted to receive care in HMOs, a recent article found young medical students willing to work in such settings and more comfortable with the projected loss of income and decreased autonomy.

Clearly, the jury is still out on attitudes of new physicians toward managed care and specifically toward HMOs, but, as the proportion of women entering medical school stabilizes at about 42 percent, certain aspects of this kind of practice, such as predictable hours and reasonable call schedules, might hold considerable appeal.

How, then, can health care providers work most productively in this kind of setting? Perhaps the most important point is that no two HMOs are alike. Like other organizations, they span the range from poorly managed, poor quality, financially troubled to well managed, high-quality organizations with sound financial bases. Some, such as Kaiser Permanente, own their own clinics, hospitals, and ancillary services, and clinicians in group practices spend full time serving enrollees, sharing a cohesive culture and willingly abiding by shared guidelines. Others depend on a range of community physicians and facilities, with doctors responsible for a mix of fee-for-service patients and enrollees from a variety of programs, each group often being "managed" according to a different set of rules. In addition, plans vary in their histories; the programs they provide; the ideologies of their managers; their profit orientations; and, perhaps most important, in the vision they have of what care should and must be for their patients.

It should be no surprise that there is large variation in styles of practice, in use of resources, and consequently in patient and provider satisfaction. This scenario is made even more complicated by the lack of shared and articulated knowledge about what works and what doesn't. Given the uncertainties of much of medical care, it is inevitable that utilization management, practiced by all HMOs, will result in denial of some care that might be beneficial. It has been shown repeatedly, in health care as well as in other industries, that incentives work remarkably well. If the operating style of the organization is to maximize profits at the expense of other values, such techniques as withholding remuneration from primary care physicians and penalizing those who fail to stay within utilization targets are likely to be used.[17]

Remarkably, HMO penetration varies so widely from one part of the country to another and can change so abruptly from almost no penetration to significant penetration that the practice environment can be dramatically different from one month to the next, leaving some health care providers wondering why their waiting rooms are so empty and others wondering how they can begin to provide care that is consistent with unfamiliar practice guidelines and a morass of referral forms. Some HMOs, for example, are predicting a dramatic decrease in hospital utilization and have come close to eliminating the need for all but the most intensive care. As this trend continues, there is an overall movement toward providing as much care as possible in an ambulatory setting, which is sometimes less costly.

As these trends continue, the percentage of the total health care dollar spent in the hospital declines dramatically, with corresponding increases in the percentage spent on physician and other services. In the 1970s, approximately 60 to 70 percent of the health care dollar was spent on hospital care; in this decade the hospital share has decreased to 25 to 30 percent. Conversely, the amount of the health care dollar spent on physician services has gone from 30 to 40 percent in the 1970s to 70 percent today. Resources will be available to reimburse health care providers, particularly primary care practitioners, for their cognitive and patient management skills if those skills continue to prove valuable to the health care system as a whole. In this regard, HMOs are already shifting an increasing portion of the health care premium dollar from subspecialists to primary care physicians in order to recognize the cognitive nature and the value of the primary care physician's skills.

The obvious lack of balance between supply and demand bodes well for primary care physicians during the coming decade and less well for certain specialists and subspecialists who will be in surplus supply during the latter part of the 1990s as the volume of services being referred to subspecialists per 1,000 population continues to decrease, further aggravating the surplus supply problem. Multispecialty groups have already begun to respond to this market reality, dramatically altering the mix of physician members. Studies are already suggesting, however, that, for many diagnoses, immediate referral to a specialist may result in a higher quality of care as well as a cost savings.

The issue of "management" is a complex one. How are patients to be managed? What does patient management actually mean? Does it refer to a practitioner who makes informed judgments of what a patient needs and manages the patient to ensure an appropriate pattern of care? Or does it simply mean a tool for controlling costs and utilization, with less attention to patient needs? Tensions exist between allocation of services and limitations of a fixed payment. As an increasing number of lives become "fully capitated, placing HMOs even more at risk, these tensions will increase rather than decrease.

Steps are being taken to decrease the uncertainty that characterizes so much of medical care. Research, collectively known as outcomes research, may shed light on the area between the need to function under some kind of budgeted arrangement and the need for the physician to remain an advocate for the patient. With better information about treatment efficacy, there are of course legitimate ways that managed care approaches can provide high-quality economical care. Lewis Thomas, in *Lives of a Cell,* tells a story about his father, a general practitioner who had few diagnostic tools at his disposal and yet had enjoyed a remarkable degree of loyalty and trust from his patients. Thomas noted that, today, a physician is far more likely to make an accurate diagnosis and to treat a condition appropriately and yet enjoy far less devotion. The issue of devotion and trust is complex and is embedded in a host of changed cultural norms that are beyond the goals of this chapter. Yet the issue of knowledge, its use and its dissemination, is not. Considerably more data exist than are, in fact, shared and used. Outcomes research may provide the necessary bridge between fee-for-service medicine and intelligently practiced managed care by shedding light on what should not be done because it is unlikely to have the desired effect and on what might be attempted even in the face of poor odds.

Perhaps alternative and sometimes less expensive services might substitute well for expensive technical approaches that sometimes yield few benefits. In fact, simple solutions, such as substitution of some nursing time for some physician time, may result in a better solution for the patient than an additional and costly test. However, such changes will only be considered and will only work if the overall incentive structure of the HMO encourages effective care rather than short-term profit. In reality, such changes are likely to take place far more readily in situations where capitation is the underlying mechanism of payment.

Conclusions

Managed care has become the buzzword of the decade and is used so widely and in so many different ways that, to a great extent, it has lost all meaning. HMOs started out with the highest of ideals: to provide comprehensive care for a specific population and to do so in one place, offering both convenience and quality. For many people, the connotation today of the HMO is that of "quick and dirty medicine," devoid of quality and, perhaps more seriously, of dignity and caring.

Whether or not public acceptance this unfortunate definition continues and grows will largely depend on the role of health care providers, because ultimately, regardless of controls and incentives, it will be clinicians who provide care and make decisions. The stance of the group of physicians described earlier in the chapter, who refused to look beyond the present and insisted on reaffirming the past, is not useful.

The health system is in the process of restructuring and of major reform. Employers will continue to play a dominant role in this process as they recognize the effect that an out-of-control health delivery system will have on profits and long-term viability. Health care providers and health administrators must learn about possible alternative structures, including the well-managed HMO. They must learn to assess how one plan differs from another, including the values of the senior decision makers, the programs they provide, the quality of personnel they enlist, the accepted managerial style, and the degree to which the profit motive coexists with attention to the needs of patients.

Just as the clinician needs to play a far more active role in the process of care delivery, the patient must take increased responsibility for his or her own health. Once again, the practitioner must lead the effort. As one physician said recently, "If one of my diabetic patients ends up in the emergency department, it is at least partly my failure." Patient education and development of a partnership between the patient and the health care provider within the context of a managed care organization represent the kind of health delivery system that will meet societal needs. This system will be characterized by providers who are operating within a controlled environment, with some level of utilization review and some form of clinical guidelines and protocols determined by ongoing outcomes research, but who are strong advocates for their patients. Clinicians should feel responsible for advocating for their patients' interests when they have a basis for believing that these interests are being slighted. To the extent that a health care provider feels that necessary care is being denied, he or she has an obligation to inform the patient. This level of advocacy will have considerably more weight in situations where the provider understands the care delivery system as a whole, including the tensions that will continue to exist between the competitive needs of the HMO and the needs of the patient.

To a great extent, the easy changes have already occurred within the managed care arena. Savings to date have largely been achieved by lowering the length of stay through utilization review and case management. In the current generation of managed care, the emphasis is on deciding what care should be provided and in what setting. Ultimately, managed care will have to build on these early efforts and integrate finance, administration, and delivery. It will encompass profiling and quality measures and decisions concerning the best mix of outpatient and inpatient care, often blurring the somewhat artificial boundaries between the two. The result will be a tightly managed, coordinated care network, with physicians continuing to play the key roles. Along the way, the expected tensions will result in a host of delivery problems as "ideals" are considered, attempted, and rejected.

A good example is the obstetric patient. What was a routine three-day hospital stay a decade ago has been drastically reduced to a day or sometimes less than a day. A host of complications are causing new debate and will in all likelihood result in new guidelines and definitions for this level of care. For every diagnosis and treatment there will be debate, but it must be the health care provider who plays the key decision-making role.

References

1. "The State of Health Care in America." *Business and Health* 13(3,Suppl C):24, 1995.
2. Roberts, M. *Your Money or Your Life. The Health Care Crisis Explained.* New York, N.Y.: Doubleday, 1993, p. 44.
3. "The State of Health Care in America." *Business and Health* 12(3,Suppl A):4-66, 1994.
4. Manning, W., and others. "A Controlled Trial of the Effect of a Prepaid Group Practice on Use of Services." *New England Journal of Medicine* 310(23):1505-10, June 7, 1984.
5. Miller, H., and Luft, H. "Managed Care Plan Performance since 1980." *JAMA* 271(19):1512-8, May 18, 1994.
6. Robinson, J. "HMO Market Penetration and Hospital Cost Inflation in California." *JAMA* 266(19):2719-23, Nov. 20, 1991.

7. Bernstein, A., and others. "Differences in Rates of Cancer Screening by Usual Source of Medical Care: Data from the 1987 National Health Interview Survey." *Medical Care* 29(3):196-209, March 1991.

8. Hellinger, F. "Selection Bias in HMOs and PPOs. A Review of the Evidence." *Inquiry* 32(2):135-42, Summer 1995.

9. Enthoven, A. "Why Managed Care Has Failed to Contain Health Costs." *Health Affairs* 12(3):27-43, Fall 1993.

10. Staines, V. "Impact of Managed Care on National Health Spending." *Health Affairs* 12(Suppl):248-57, 1993.

11. Fox., H., and others. "Health Maintenance Organizations and Children with Special Health Needs." *American Journal of Diseases of Children* 147(5):546-52, May 1993.

12. Wooley, S. "Managed Care and Mental Health: the Silencing of a Profession." *International Journal of Eating Disorders* 14(4):387-401, Dec. 1993.

13. Davis, K., and others. "Choice Matters: Enrollees' Views of Their Health Plans." *Health Affairs* 14(2):102-11, Summer 1995.

14. Rubin, H. "Patients' Ratings of Outpatient Visits in Different Practice Settings." *JAMA* 270(7):835-40, Aug. 18, 1993.

15. Garnick, D., and others. "How Well Do American Understand Their Health Coverage?" *Health Affairs* 12(3):204-12, Fall 1993.

16. Schulz, R. "Physician Satisfaction in a Managed Care Environment." *Journal of Family Practice* 34(3):298-304, March 1992.

17. Mechanic, D. "Managed Care: Rhetoric and Realities." *Inquiry* 31(2):124-28, Summer 1994

Diana Barrett, DBA, is Lecturer in Management, Harvard School of Public Health, Boston, Massachusetts.

Chapter 4

Independent Practice Association Model of Managed Care

by Budd N. Shenkin, MD, MAPA

The structure of the health care system was for decades like a frozen river, seemingly solid and immobile, with only an occasional crack visible at the surface. Now the ice pack has suddenly broken up and begun to flow down river with such speed and violence that large chunks of it will doubtless be lurching and crashing into each other. For a while, it looked as though the new structure would be controlled by new government rules of the river. Now it seems clear that "natural" market rules of free flow are to prevail. With such dynamism set loose, we have to expect that the structures and connections we observe today might well bear little resemblance to the final result, although these early structures and the efforts we make now will surely condition the structure of the (ideally) more tranquil future.

Let me abandon the metaphor at this point, hoping that it conveys the picture of rapid health care institutional change and the unlikelihood of early resolution. My assignment in this chapter is to explain and make the case for one of the early entities produced by managed care, the independent practice association (IPA) model. This I will do with some enthusiasm, because I believe that IPAs give physicians the best opportunity available to assemble a new and workable health care system with themselves as active participants in setting policy. Even if IPAs turn out to be only transitional structures, they will confer to future structures a salubrious relationship between the system and health care providers.

To make the case properly, I will not only describe the IPA model, but also try to place IPAs in the perspective of the general movement of the health care market and institutions and identify issues of enduring concern. I will address the following questions:

- Can we expect managed care to produce an improved system of care?
- What do providers want and need from the new system of care?
- What types of managed care organizations are extant?

- How can we compare and contrast managed care models?
- What are the critical variables of IPA organization?
- What will competition look like in local areas?
- Who will control what aspects of the health care system?

What Are the Prospects of Managed Care?

Because managed care was produced explicitly to reduce costs, it is easy to be cynical in assessing its prospects for improving the system and maintaining quality. If we look at reforms in other industries, however, the evidence shows that better, more productive systems have been instituted primarily in response to similar problems of cost control.[1] Bloated as it is with inefficiencies, the medical care system should be no different.

But to say that something is possible is not to say that it is easy. Success in managed care will hinge on how it will be done, and who will do it. A key factor will be: What role will health care providers take in designing and implementing managed care, and what will their role be in its functioning? Mindless resistance by providers will be counterproductive, but involvement simply to retain the wasteful patterns of the past will be just as bad. Health care providers are intelligent participants and observers of the health care system; if they sincerely involve themselves with some degree of "can-do" spirit, the eventual system could be markedly superior to the previous one.

What Do Physicians Want and Need?

Many goals of health care providers are ones that patients will share. After all, a well-functioning industry serves clients, workers, and owners better than one that functions poorly; it is not a zero-sum game.

Some believe, of course, that health care providers merely want to protect their incomes. Of course, that is one of our objectives. Altruistic we may be, but we continue to live in a capitalistic society where money counts, for attaining material and other goals as well as social prestige. Different providers get there at different rates of speed, but most eventually want to do well in return for doing good. Many patients share this objective for providers, by the way, although perhaps not with the same intensity. If providers are not well compensated, how enthusiastically will they function, and who will aspire to become one?

But to think that money is our sole objective is naïve.[2] We need medicine to be professionally rewarding, even if we must adopt the business orientation that a capitalistic economy demands. We need to preserve our medical ethic, putting the patient first, practicing beneficence and truth in communications, pursuing scientific objectivity, working hard, and maintaining personal connections with our patients and their progress. Medical ethics need to predominate over business ethics. We need to make sure that our reformed organizations work, that they are rational and efficient, not crazily bureaucratic nor insanely entrepreneurial. We need a variety of organizational choices to be available, because both physicians and patients come in a variety of personalities, some functioning well in small units, others in larger ones, some tolerant of risk, others craving security. We need to make sure that organizations are fair to all physicians, individually, while the public interest is protected. As the archetypes of autonomous professionals, we need to be able to feel like doctors, not like general contractors, bureaucrats, or (sad to say) public school teachers.

The Types of Managed Care Organizations

In this early evolution of managed care organizations, three basic models seem to have emerged at the regional level (see figure below). The first model is the so-called integrated health plan. In one version of this model, the Kaiser model, the physician group is organized as a discreet entity. Other integrated plans employ physicians as individuals rather than as a group.

Models of Managed Care

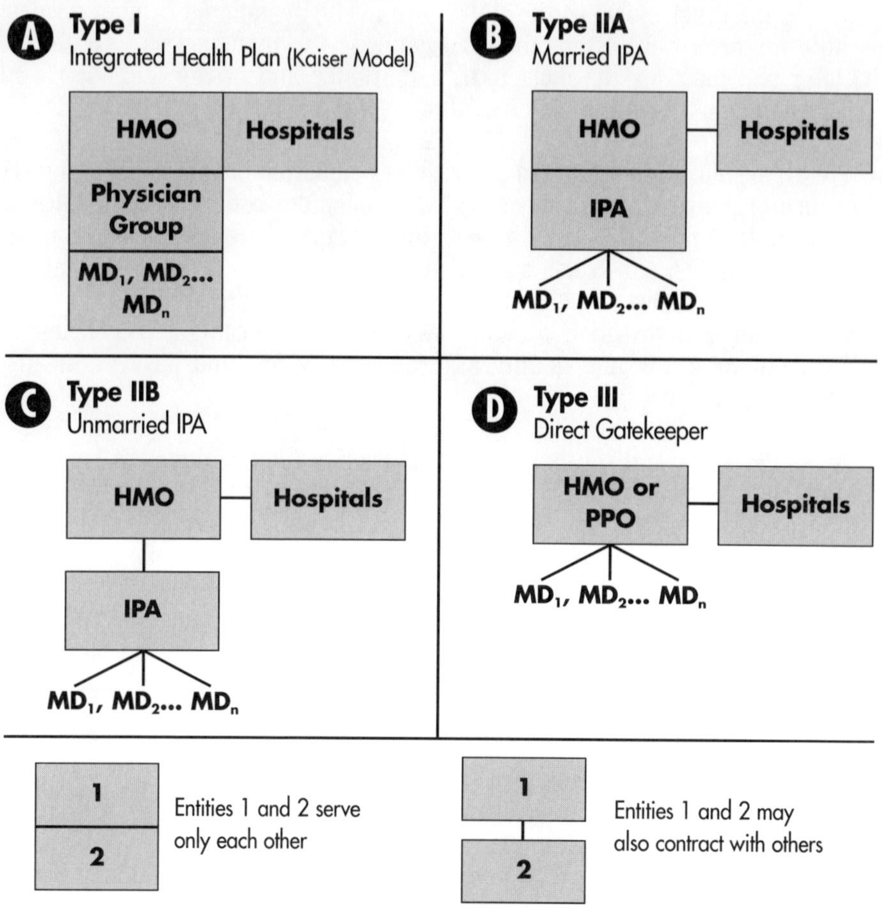

At the other extreme of organization is the so-called direct gatekeeper model of managed care. In this model, insurance companies (or HMOs) contract directly with individual providers to service their products.

In-between the extremes of these two models is the IPA model. IPAs come in two basic varieties, "married" and "unmarried." The married IPA relates to its one and only HMO; neither is tempted (presumably) even to flirt with other organizations for their services. The unmarried variety, conversely, can hold many contracts and serve many different plans. IPA physicians and integrated health plan physicians present a very different organizational front to the patient: the former look like private practitioners, using their own offices and serving patients other than HMO patients, whereas a Kaiser physician, for example, works in a Kaiser building and sees only Kaiser patients.

It can be confusing to try to distinguish the basic functions of HMOs and IPAs. The HMO sits between payers and providers, marketing the plan and setting benefits and premiums on the one hand, and contracting with IPAs and hospitals to deliver the care on the other. Because the HMO pays mostly negotiated capitated rates, it runs little financial risk. After initially organizing the managed care system, the HMO later becomes, for the most part, a marketer and broker, although it also aspires, as a buyers' agent, to be an evaluator of IPA services.

The IPA, an organization of physicians, receives capitated payments from the HMO and in turn organizes the delivery of care. It concludes contracts with HMOs and PPOs; assembles, credentials, and inspects the network of provider physicians, institutions, and services; constructs authorization and referral processes; establishes gatekeeper and specialist responsibilities, sometimes including treatment protocols; disburses payment to providers and ancillary services according to its policies; conducts utilization review and quality assurance activities; and ensures the fiscal integrity of the enterprise.

IPAs make decisions and set policies that determine the conditions of health care providers' professional lives. They decide on such crucial issues as physician membership, practice policies, and distribution of money. They decide the patients a physician has access to; policies on scope of practice and gatekeeping; reimbursement methods and amounts; the list of physicians, therapists, hospitals, laboratories, and emergency facilities that physicians can refer to; and methods of referral and authorization. They have access to office records for audit and can enforce standards of care and access offered to the public. No entity in medicine has had such power heretofore over independently practicing physicians.

Compare and Contrast the Three Models

The above typology forms an organizational spectrum stretching from physicians amalgamated into a very large bureaucratic scheme without practice autonomy on the one hand, to isolated individual practitioners without a group relationship on the other. In theory, the IPA model may have substantial advantages over both extremes.

Large, Integrated Systems versus IPAs

The Kaiser system has been well accepted by many patients and physicians, and some say that economies of scale will force all medicine into such large scale systems. Large organizations, however, are not inherently more cost-efficient than small practices. Prior to managed care, it was widely believed that optimal efficiency lay in groups of four to six physicians. Furthermore, the nonmedical world of large corporations has tried to reduce scale for the sake of efficiency, and decentralization with the creation of artificial profit centers has been a trend for decades.[3] Experienced observers of medical group practices believe that larger organizations may try to replicate many of the qualities of small-scale practices, but their size and bureaucratic complexity are always working against them.[4] It is true that large groups have shown survivability superior to small groups and individual practices, and that the "managed care industry" aims for groups of 25-30 providers, but this may well be due to power in the marketplace and other nonefficiency criteria.[5]

In terms of personal responsiveness, a small practice cannot be rivaled by a large integrated plan. Small and understandable scale, with repetitive personal interactions with known personnel, is a virtue in itself to many patients and physicians. Many physicians express their creativity by organizing and running their practices in their own way. Many work better under conditions in which they palpably profit from their own work and intelligence. It is far from unreasonable for a physician to want to control his or her own office, to hire and fire staff members, to direct their functioning, and to reap the profit that comes as a reward—and many patients prefer it that way, too. Many physicians are eager to continue as direct participants in the capitalistic system, which they may regard as the "means for efficiency and freedom."[6]

The idea of the IPA model is to preserve small practices and to graft onto them larger scale management functions at the IPA level.

Direct Gatekeeper Model versus IPAs

At the other pole of the spectrum, direct gatekeeper advocates argue that IPAs simply add another bureaucratic layer to the system. The direct gatekeeper model, however, relying on top-down and nonparticipatory regulatory authority, is simply too distant from practitioners to reconfigure patterns of care. It can only exhort participants with "Letters from the Director," increase surveillance of care with annoying 1-800 numbers, and change fees and allowed procedures without consultation. In this model, any arbitrary steps taken by the plan cannot be countermanded by physicians, because they contract as individuals rather than as a unified group.

The real task of managed care is to invent and develop cost-saving patterns of care, changing reimbursement, work incentives, and culture of care for both primary care physicians and specialists. IPAs provide the sort of organization that can facilitate change. As currently structured, they are small and decentralized enough to foster reiterative personal exchanges at the operational level as information is received and new procedures are introduced.[7] The group of peers forming an IPA should be able to provide intellectual stimulation, emotional support, and personal reality testing for their leadership in a situation of change. While accommodations to the group will need to be made, the IPA should enable providers to retain a strong sense of autonomy. If properly led, IPAs should ensure that physician ethics rather than business ethics, and physician knowledge rather than administrator knowledge of the implications of medical decisions, will guide decisions.

Take a simple technical (rather than political) example. Suppose a national study calls for decisive changes in the outpatient treatment of diabetes. If the call were for inpatient changes, the hospital committee system could probably handle implementation. But how will outpatient changes be implemented? By having an insurance company send out letters to its thousands of individual contractors, declaring a new insurance company reimbursement policy, so physicians will now be reimbursed only if they do things a certain way? That is risible. The locally based IPA, with its ability to have physicians mull over decisions and procedure changes, should be an institution made to order for effecting these progressive changes.

Many of the tasks of reform, however, are more political than technical, involving issues of money, conditions of work for health care providers, and relations among different constituent groups. For instance, most IPAs face the need to modify the severe income discrepancies between primary care practitioners and the procedural specialists. In theory, the IPA should be able to accomplish a political-economic mission that the other models cannot. Direct gatekeeper physicians have no unified voice, and integrated plan physicians, as employees or near-employees, may well need union representation, with the possible proletarianization and loss of professionalism that that implies. Unlike the other two models, IPAs—created by local initiatives, self-governing in principle, and with entirely local membership—offer the possibility of participation in management instead of unionization, and "bottom-up" influence to counter "top-down" pressure.

The Critical Variables of IPA Organization

New organizations are subject to invention, innovation, a high effort-to-result ratio, and failure. Current IPAs exhibit all those characteristics.

Forms of Organization and Funding

Although the IPA is, in principle, an organization of physicians, organizing and funding such a complex organization is difficult and expensive, so that physicians can easily be tempted to rely on others for sponsorship of the IPA. The most traditional source of such support is the local hospital, which, unlike physicians, is accustomed to retaining funds for investment and organizing ventures. Hospitals have proved quite willing to organize and fund IPAs, because they understand that IPAs and "covered lives" are necessary for their own continued existence. Their progressive renaming of themselves from "hospitals" to "medical centers" to "health systems" reveals their vision. The problem, of course, is that relying on a hospital to build and maintain an IPA inevitably constrains that IPA's future vision and action. Other choices are available for support and partnership: regional or national IPAs are willing to "affiliate" with a local group; HMOs will themselves construct IPAs of the "married" type; national firms now exist to construct and run IPAs. There is no such thing as a free lunch: the more a group of physicians relies on its own money and own efforts, the more it will be free to plot its own destiny and make alliances in the marketplace with its own welfare in mind.

The IPA must also decide on its basic form of organization. If it has been able to remain independent, the most dynamic American institution, the business corporation, recommends itself. The IPA is not exactly like most corporations, of course, because physician members are usually shareholders and funders of the organization. Thus, they are not employees, and they are not exactly independent contractors, either. But other models of organization with which physicians are familiar (the co-op, the medical staff, the county medical organization) would seem unsuited for the dynamism necessary for the IPA. If it does elect the corporate form, the IPA will have to invent mechanisms to adapt that form to the fact that ownership is widespread among the member physicians.

If physicians are not able to achieve independence, they may find themselves with a hospital within a physician hospital organization (PHO) or even as a subdivision of an HMO. In either case, physicians will share power with an entity whose interests are at variance with theirs and that, as a unified institution, has strong advantages over physicians in deciding policy.

Administrative Leadership

The seemingly simple act of settling on an administrative structure and finding personnel to run the technical side of the operation will often be daunting. Initially, the IPA must be constructed, which means establishing a network of physician providers and negotiating contracts with hospital and ancillary providers, deciding upon reimbursement techniques, setting up a system to track and pay claims, ensuring fiscal solvency, controlling utilization and quality, and then negotiating and securing contracts with HMOs and PPOs. Accomplishing these basic tasks is technically and politically difficult.

While physicians will want to be in charge of IPA policy, they will also want to remain in practice. Yet full-time attention is necessary for such a group. Even if a physician wants to quit practice and administer full time, he or she would typically lack the proper training and would be suspected by peers of self-aggrandizement. (On the other hand, it is important for an organization to find a way to reward its leaders according to their contributions, which will typically exceed those of the bulk of the organization.) Physician leaders need to be able to guide the ship without doing the steering themselves. Finding physician leadership that can walk this tightrope is crucial.

Trained and experienced administrators are necessary, but finding administrators with a profound understanding of the health care system who are able to organize company operations, to deal effectively with both physicians and HMO administrators, and to be entrepreneurial is not an easy job. Finding a way for new organizations to attract and retain them is harder still. Finding such persons, who paradoxically value an organization that empowers physicians and limits their own power as administrators, would seem to be a rare event. Because IPAs are new types of organizations, finding administrators with relevant experience will be difficult. In fact, the difficulty of this task will no doubt be a key limiting factor in IPA proliferation around the country.

Freedom versus Authority

IPAs require firm leadership because many difficult and unpleasant tasks must be accomplished—for example, telling proceduralists that they will have to make less money, and exerting group control over individual patterns of practice. The corporate model can support firm leadership.

But what is the place of health care providers in a corporate model? Relating businesses to professionals is always difficult, even when the relationship is clearly that of employer and employee.[8] Businesses usually deal either with employees inside the organization or with contractors and suppliers providing services from outside the organization. IPA physicians are clearly not employees. But are they merely contractors for services? Professionals who ensure the trust of the public in the entire enterprise and who hold themselves to standards unlike those in virtually any other line of endeavor are clearly more than traditional contractors and suppliers. In fact, according to one observer, only the physicians' professional medical ethic will enable managed care to work, if it can.[9] Moreover, it is these physicians who established the IPA and who hold shares in it.

If the IPA is governed by a corporate board, to what extent must that board present its policies to the membership and be elected on that basis? If such membership pressure is present, to what extent is leadership impeded? Will the IPA be able to dismiss members without cause, thus strengthening the authority of the IPA at the expense of member freedom? Are members required to serve exclusively with one IPA, thus sacrificing their leverage on the policies of that IPA as well as their individual practice potential and safety (for instance, if the IPA fails) for the welfare of the group? Finding a way to honor the need for authority and still to acknowledge the needs of providers for autonomy may constitute the most difficult political problem of these new organizations.

The Ultimate Goal of the Organization

Ultimately, the IPA will have to arrive at a vision shared by leaders and members. IPAs begin as a mechanism to allow constituent providers to continue in decentralized, independently owned physician practices. Once established, however, the IPA will inevitably enjoy a new perspective. All of a sudden, a group more cohesive than an IPA will look more attractive and become more feasible, as health care providers settle into these organizations and establish informal alliances. An initially successful IPA can be inspired to think (or an IPA under severe competitive pressure might be constrained to think) that it can expand and provide such good care in an area that it will become predominant. By doing so, the IPA would earn the right to deal with large HMOs on a more equal footing.

Can the advantages of a more cohesive group outweigh the inevitable increase in bureaucratic friction, change of culture, and decrease in autonomy? If a size increase is planned, would it blunt the very advantages of small groups that IPAs promise? At precisely this point, one would think, the organizational decision-making process would become paramount. If the rank and file do not have a vigorous voice in the organization, the decision to become more integrated could be more a threat than an invitation.

Competitive Structure in a Regional Area

In addition to an IPA's internal structure, the milieu in which an IPA exists will exert an important effect. For example, primary care providers and specialists will enjoy increased leverage if they have alternative IPAs to which they could potentially switch their allegiance. Under the common conditions of excess physician supply, some health care providers will want to control an IPA and to keep competitors out. IPAs themselves will want few competitors. They will wish to lock up their physicians, denying them the freedom to switch, and thus be able to face HMOs, hopefully many of them, with a unique product as an established force in the area. They will also want to establish exclusive contracts with HMOs to freeze potential competitors out. HMOs will prefer either a married IPA that it can control, or several overlapping IPAs from which to choose, with few or no other competing HMOs. Purchasers will prefer a wide choice of overlapping HMOs. All participants will do what they can to bring about whichever of these or other favorable conditions they can.

The ideal competitive structure in a local or regional area is not immediately obvious. Despite their desire for choice and competition among suppliers, which often implies smallness, participants will want fully elaborated products and organizational stability, characteristics of larger organizational entities. Also, as Schumpeter observed, larger sized corporations more commonly compete on the basis of technologic and organizational innovation rather than simply of price.[10] In addition, industrial innovation is generally aided if there is enough challenge in the environment to be invigorating, but enough security to be able to take a chance. An IPA should ideally not have the field to itself, but it should not be so threatened that it may be pushed to extinction with one mistake. Still, observations of events in small areas with strong IPA competition do reveal that rapid technologic innovation can occur in the context of sharp IPA competition.[11]

The structure of regional competition has obviously not yet been played out, even in mature areas. In America, we usually let early competition structure a market and then let government observe the results and propose corrective market regulation to foster "fair competition." In the case of managed care, however, the private movement is so fast that governmental forces appear to be far behind even in understanding the present, let alone analyzing the future and proposing corrective measures.

From observations at one local level, it appears that free entry of IPAs to the field, a key component of fully functioning free market competition, is not met.[11] When a few large IPAs have been formed in an area and HMO contracts are secured, the HMOs have not extended further contracts to potentially competing IPAs. Consequently, when physicians from the county medical society, or physicians leaving one IPA to form their own, or health care providers not included in the current large IPAs want to form their own IPA and compete, they cannot get contracts. If they could, such new additions might contribute organizational innovations, give a hope of continuing to practice to currently excluded health care providers, and certainly add discipline to current market players. A proliferation of IPAs would also enable any single IPA to exercise more control over its members without encountering criticism, because member providers could always move to another IPA if they chose.

To alleviate this market fault, I have proposed a legislative remedy called "Any Willing IPA."[12] This legislation would require an HMO that has contracted with any IPA in a regional area to contract at similar terms with any willing (and qualified) IPA also serving that area.

A second market fault appears to be excessive HMO advantage in negotiating with IPAs and payers, resulting in apparently excessive HMO profits. The current trend of HMO consolidation will only make this condition more severe. Because the "single payer" alternative has been voted down in the U.S. Congress and in California, government regulation is the obvious next candidate for control. These and other government remedies to aid fair competition should be considered as we judge how best to structure competition within areas.

Who Will Control the Health Care System?

Before managed care, one "radical" view was that physicians controlled the health care system as "professional monopolists," but that they would soon be challenged by "corporate rationalizers," such as hospitals, planners, and insurance companies.[13] Managed care certainly seems to be the vehicle for that institutional challenge. As agglomeration proceeds, the question of who controls health care will be decided by the nature of the participant organizations, who controls each one, and what their relations are with one another.

To participate in the game, physicians clearly must agglomerate. Even though IPAs may be transitory organizations, they have the virtue of being provider-based. Politically, they may be just what health care providers need as leadership and organizational experience among providers is developed. The corporate rationalizers are certainly right when they say that the health care system must be reorganized. Still, any such reorganization will also entail a change in who controls what part and how much of the system.

There are system rationalization goals to be accomplished, and there are political goals of self-determination and autonomy. It may well be in the interest of health care providers to perpetuate the division between the insurance and marketing functions, currently ensconced at the HMO and insurance company level, and the organization and delivery of care functions, situated at the IPA level. Separation would enable insurance and marketing entities to concentrate on their functions while the medical care entities would concentrate on theirs. The medical profession would be responsible to itself and to the market, not directly to a business authority with an agenda to exert control over the whole system.

References

1. Stymne, B. "Reorganization of Work: Causes and Effects." In Rinnooy, K., Editor, *New Challenges for Management Research.* North-Holland: Elsevier Science Publishers, 1985, pp. 93-113, 102-103.
2. Lane, R. *The Market Experience.* Cambridge, England: Cambridge University Press, 1991.
3. Williamson, O. *Corporate Control and Business Behavior.* Englewood Cliffs, N.J.: Prentice-Hall, 1970.
4. Donald L. Madison, MD, Professor of Social Medicine, University of North Carolina, Chapel Hill, personal communication.
5. Schiff, M. Medical Group Practice: *A Survivor Analysis from 1969 to 1991.* Unpublished master's degree thesis, University of California, Berkeley, 1993.
6. Heilbroner, R. *The Nature and Logic of Capitalism.* New York, N.Y.: W.W. Norton, 1985, p. 151.
7. Lewin, K. "Group Decision and Social Change." In Maccoby, E., and others, Editors, *Readings in Social Psychology, 3rd Edition,* New York, N.Y.: Holt, Rinehart and Winston, 1958, pp. 197-211.
8. Etzioni, A. *Modern Organizations.* Englewood Cliffs, N.J.: Prentice-Hall, 1964, pp. 75-8.
9. Blumenthal, D. "The Vital Role of Professionalism in Health Care Reform." *Health Affairs* 13(1):252-6, Spring (I) 1994.
10. Schumpeter, J., and Bottome, T. *Capitalism, Socialism, and Democracy.* New York, N.Y.: Harper & Row, 1993.
11. Shenkin, B. "The Independent Practice Association in Theory and Practice: Lessons from Experience." *JAMA* 273(24):1937-42, June 28, 1995.
12. Shenkin, B. "Any Willing IPA: Shaping the Market through Legislation." *American Journal of Managed Care,* May 1996, pp. 524-31.
13. Shenkin, B. "The Liberals Aren't the Good Guys, Either: A Review Essay on Health Care Politics: Ideological and Interest Group Barriers to Reform by Robert A Alford. *Journal of Community Health* 2(3):232-41, Spring 1977.

Budd N. Shenkin, MD, MAPA, is Executive Director, Center for Responsive Health Policy, Berkeley, California.

Chapter 5

Overview of Physician Hospital Organizations and Physician Organizations

by Eileen Weis, MSHA, and Kimball Austin Miller, MD, MSHA

Introduction

The provision of health care is changing rapidly because of limited government and corporate resources and the rapid growth of managed care. Physicians and hospitals are revamping the way in which they conduct business. As in any industry experiencing structural and elemental widespread change, opportunities are plentiful to create the future environment. Physicians and hospitals are discovering that, by forming partnerships, they can shape a future that is both energizing and favorable, not only for themselves but also for their communities.

A physician hospital organization (PHO) represents the first step in working together toward a better future in the managed care environment. The organization seeks to preserve the provider-patient relationship while managing it. This overview will describe the physician hospital organization structure, organizational development process, capitalization models, organizational management issues, and predictors of success.

Physician Hospital Organization Structures

The PHO creates a structure in which separate businesses, one or more hospitals and physicians, come together to participate in managed care. The PHO's main purpose is to be a cost-efficient contracting entity for its owners, not a financial mechanism for returning dividends to its investors/owners.

PHO development is usually initiated by a hospital. Hospitals are redefining their role in the health care system by teaming with physicians in PHOs. PHOs create an introductory structure for hospitals and physicians to learn together about risk sharing; medical management, including credentialing, provider selection, utilization management, quality assurance, formulary management, health promotion, demand management, outcome measurement, relationship management, and grievance abatement; and cost control. As providers experience success in a discounted fee-for-service managed care environment, they will gain confidence to move into a higher risk contract setting that necessitates greater integration, resource utilization review, and capitation.

Many observers believe that PHOs are a short-term phenomenon and will gradually be replaced by more formal, contract-bound, integrated structures that are better equipped to reduce costs and improve quality of care. In an evolving managed care market, the PHO is usually the first step in a continuum of business structures that progressively move providers into risk-sharing ventures:

- Traditional fee-for-service arrangement.
- Loose alliance of providers, with imposition of reasonable and customary payment limits and discounts.
- Increasing consolidation of services, with provider risk pools, some medical management, and withholding.
- Advanced, fully integrated delivery systems, with capitation and ability to provide and manage the complete continuum of care.[1]

The PHO is often the transitional structure for moving providers from a traditional fee-for-service environment to a setting that has some consolidation and can effectively handle limited risk. Within the PHO structure, providers have a lot of latitude in the degree of integration, amount of medical management or operational control, and risk that they want to adopt. Most of them begin as loosely affiliated entities, with the intention of converting to more closely knit structures over time.

PHOs generally advance through three evolutionary phases. First-generation PHOs are typically specialty-dominated or sometimes hospital-dominated. They are the most politically safe form of organization. The physician panel is open to virtually the entire medical staff, with no provider selection or reappointment mechanisms in place that account for utilization of resources or quality of care performance. Payment for service is usually on a discounted fee-for-service basis. Controls for profitably handling risk contracting are absent. Managed care intermediaries are usually charged with conducting utilization management (prior authorization, concurrent review, case management, and utilization review), quality assurance, formulary management, outcome measurement, and credentialing.

Research has documented that PHO structures that stay in the first stage are too loose in medical management to survive financially over the long term. Without some of the more sophisticated and expensive utilization review, quality assurance, and operations management systems in place, these PHOs are unable to tightly monitor resource usage, quality, and costs. Many of these PHOs are unwilling or unable to invest in organizational management infrastructures, including sophisticated information systems. Physicians and hospitals continue to bill separately for services, operating solely on a discounted fee-for-service basis. Local payers and/or community employers prefer this simple discounted fee-for-service arrangement over more traditional and expensive full fee-for-service payment structures. In these situations, the PHO looks more like a simple IPA, except that it has a hospital member. Such PHOs, found in rural areas, can operate successfully in this environment because of the low number of provider options and the limited amount of managed care in their markets.

The third-generation PHO is the most advanced, in that it is an integrated management entity with consolidation of some resources. Primary care physicians dominate the governance structures, are usually the formal and/or informal leaders, and constitute at least 40 percent of the physician panel. These PHOs share risk fully among hospitals and physicians in the provision of managed care. They typically invest in comprehensive information systems, employ national credentialing standards, use efficient in-house utilization management and quality assurance programs, and conduct performance-based appointment of physicians using standardized outcome measures. This entity accepts responsibility for management of all health care delivery for a specific group of capitated members without integration of all assets.

A second generation PHO is a transitional structure between the first and the third generations. In this PHO, an operational management infrastructure to manage risk is in the process of being developed. Some of the medical management functions that were previously performed by the managed care intermediary are slowly delegated to the partner organization as knowledge, skills, abilities, and funds become available to support them. This type of PHO typically covers 5,000 to 50,000 lives.[2]

Some experts advise newly developing PHOs to skip the first generation model in their development. In other words, learn from the experience of other PHOs and aggressively move forward. These new PHOs can begin by giving all health care providers medical management education, assigning key leadership and governance roles to primary care physicians, implementing strong utilization management programs, initiating quality assurance monitoring procedures, and accepting limited risk contracts and capitation reimbursement. As funds become available, they can invest in information systems that will support these PHO medical management activities.

PHOs serve a useful purpose in today's marketplace by performing the following functions for physicians and hospital providers:

- Negotiating contracts with managed care health plans and increasing patient access to managed care.
- Accepting and monitoring risk contracts.
- Preserving and managing provider assets and relationships.
- Bringing to the market innovative health care products that meet community needs, wants, and demands.
- Developing effective health promotion and risk assessment programs.
- Helping hospitals and physicians survive and prosper economically in an employer-driven managed care environment.
- Initiating case management processes that cross the entire spectrum of health care delivery.

- Linking components of health care delivery economically.
- Educating administrators and physicians about the changing health care environment.
- Developing physician leaders who are knowledgeable regarding medical management operations and cost control techniques.
- Setting community-based/specialty-determined fee schedules and age/sex capitation rates.
- Reducing bad debt by accepting capitated payments.
- Collecting data on quality indicators, outcome measures, and associated costs.
- Performing office management services that create economies of scale.
- Developing urban-nonmetropolitan health care delivery systems.[3]

Nevertheless, the PHO structure has some inherent weaknesses. Because providers usually maintain businesses that are separate from the PHO, they will continue to compete with each other in non-PHO contracts. Their previous investments of time, effort, and money in non-PHO business (i.e., solo practice office management and marketing) may diminish their motivation to fund the PHO, especially if it is viewed as a potential competitor to their traditional business.[4] Weaknesses besides those associated with limited integration include loss of some physician independence secondary to clinical practice guidelines and fixed formularies, loss of some profit because of discounted fee schedules and capitation, bureaucratic regulations and policies inherent in a PHO structure, and the administrative expense associated with building a new infrastructure.[5]

Organizational Development

Hospital Involvement in PHO Development

The success of the PHO is greatly influenced by the hospital's role in the process. A hospital that is willing to share control and decision making with physicians actively demonstrates its commitment to the PHO and to participative management. A hospital CEO who can resolve conflict constructively and has effective interpersonal skills is needed to facilitate the growth and development of the venture. The administrator who is visionary and can paint an optimistic view of the joint partnership's role in the new health care environment is an essential asset to the process.

Trust between administration and medical staff is another key ingredient to success. An administration that has earned the medical staff's trust over the years is usually more effective with physicians than is a senior staff that is relatively new to the organization. Furthermore, an administration that is part of a larger health system, such as a for-profit corporation, may have difficulty gaining the trust of physicians. Doctors can find it difficult partnering with a hospital whose major decisions are generally made on a distant corporate level. Physicians need to know that administration will make and support decisions that are good for patients, providers, and the local community.

Trust between hospital and medical staff also can be affected by a hospital's decision to purchase primary care practices. Physicians could interpret a hospital's aggressive acquisition of multiple primary care practices action as being adversarial and representing a conflict of interest with the joint venture. Hospitals that use the partnership to purchase medical and surgical practices can often assuage medical staff concerns by documenting their interest in working in a partnership format. The hospital, especially if it operates a self-funded insurance program, can demonstrate its commitment to the PHO by channeling the health benefits contract for its hospital employees to the PHO. This facilitates initiation of the joint project because it immediately provides the PHO with some managed care enrollees.

Finally, the hospital and physicians can demonstrate their commitment to the PHO by documenting a willingness to forfeit short-term financial gains for the long-term financial success of the partnership. Operating under a capitated environment will reverse incentives to generate charges. In the managed care model, the hospital and physicians are viewed as cost centers as opposed to the revenue centers they were in the previous fee-for-service, indemnity insurance system.[5]

Physician Involvement in PHO Development

Physicians' primary motivation for forming PHOs and physician organizations (POs), according to studies by the American Medical Association and medical specialty societies, is economic insecurity and the threat of change in the practice of medicine caused by the growth of managed care in their local service markets. Many physicians and hospitals that historically did not have collegial relations are suddenly interested in working together to provide health care services and to succeed in the new managed care marketplace. All partners realize that their ability to directly contract for groups of patients rests on creating and presenting a united front. Managed care is generally not a friendly environment for solo practitioners, unless they are interested in selling their practices.

The formation of a PO is crucial to the success of the PHO. If the PO has not developed prior to the PHO, physicians will often stop the PHO process until they are formally organized. Once organized, the PO can negotiate as an entity on behalf of physicians, with consensus already determined on key issues. The PO will also have the opportunity to decide if it even wants to form a PHO with the hospital.

A PO serves many useful functions for its physicians:

- Informing physicians of managed care and medical management developments.
- Developing stable provider relationships.
- Disseminating information and fostering decision making.

- Unifying physicians, which is particularly important in towns with many solo practitioners and small group partnerships.
- Presenting a united front in negotiations with hospitals.
- Enhancing contract negotiation with payers by presenting a united organizational/delivery structure.
- Reducing fear by being a proactive force that represents physician interests.[6]

Some physicians have questioned the need to develop a PO when an organized medical staff already exists. These physicians eventually learn that a PO is quite different from the traditional hospital medical staff. The medical staff tends to be dominated by specialists, is focused on inpatient care, and has expertise in determining medical staff privileges. In contrast, the PO is oriented toward primary care; is focused on managed care contracts with payers; and is keenly interested in utilization management, provider panel selection, outcome measurement, and cost reduction.

In the beginning of PHO and PO development, some overlap in medical staff and PO functions may naturally occur. For example, both entities are usually charged with performing primary source verification credentialing and quality assurance activities. To reduce duplication over the long term, some sharing of responsibilities and delegation of tasks should occur. Some people believe the PO and the medical staff will eventually merge credentialing and medical privilege activities.

Primary care physicians generally play a leading role in PHO development, determination of specialty-primary care ratios, and operations. Despite payer preferences, most PHOs are composed 30 percent of primary care physicians and 70 percent of secondary care specialists and subspecialists. Most recently surveyed PHOs have goals to increase the primary care percentage to 50 percent.[7] One option is to create a subpanel of PHO specialists to participate in some, but not all, managed care contracts. Another option is to limit the recruitment focus to primary care physicians in order to eventually achieve an even proportion of physicians. A third option is to use deselection procedures, using utilization management data and outcome measurement information, to select or retain only the most efficient specialists. The difficulty with this last option is that it can be politically undesirable. Also, many "inefficient" physicians can and will alter their practice styles, given sufficient information and time, making it difficult to reduce staff size solely on the basis of performance measures.

A PHO's success can be attributed largely to the strength of its physician leaders. These physicians generally work long and hard, navigating difficult political situations, to bring unity to the medical staff and agreement between the hospital and the PO. These physicians share several attributes:

- A clear vision of the PHO's and the PO's roles in the changing health care environment.
- Commitment to physicians and hospital working together to achieve beneficial results for all providers.
- Utilization of cooperative planning and participative management
- Understanding of the need for provider selection and annual reselection to the participating panel.
- Belief in the integrity of utilization management, quality assurance, and outcome measurement processes.
- Interest in developing creative health care delivery solutions.
- Trust and respect of the medical staff and hospital administration.

Some physicians gravitate to the leadership role because they have had previous experience in a managed care environment and have confidence in their ability to guide their peers through a similar experience. Other physicians assume leadership positions because they have previously served, or are currently serving, in leadership roles and view the PO leadership role as a natural progression. Physician leaders who devote a significant amount of time in PO and PHO development should be financially compensated on an hourly, per meeting, or capitated basis by their respective organizations. Compensation can have a significant impact on a PHO's and a PO's ability to retain high-quality physicians in leadership roles and to develop functional organizations.

Governance

Most PHOs operate under the assumption that physicians and the hospital have an equal voice. Most PHO boards reflect that preference by having an equal number of physician and hospital representatives. The PHO board, to safeguard against domination of the voting process by hospital or physician representatives, can adopt a supermajority voting provision that requires majorities of both parties before a matter is approved. Another method to ensure equal representation is to alternate the board chair position between a physician and a hospital member or to create a cochair position with one physician and one hospital representative.[8]

Community or business members can serve on the PHO Board but may or may not have voting privileges, depending on the PHO's preference. The PHO can select certain business or community members for the board, or it can appoint a nominating committee to select members so that they represent the diversity of the community. Some PHOs prefer to directly select employers who are knowledgeable about health care and represent businesses with large numbers of potential enrollees for the PHO.

Community and business members can also serve on an advisory committee that advises the board on specific matters. Some PHO boards are more comfortable having community and business representation one step away when critical matters are discussed and decided. In Atlanta, one PHO created a 14-member consumer advisory board that included insurance brokers, small business owners, and employee benefits professionals. The board assisted the PHO in developing a private-label insurance product and provided advice on financial matters, such as package pricing.[2]

Capitalization

The Federal Trade Commission strongly recommends that PHOs be funded by hospitals and physicians in a ratio that is directly proportional to their board representation. Other ratios may invite federal scrutiny for violation of antikickback rules. Regardless of the recommendations, hospitals have traditionally provided more than half, even up to 100 percent, of the capital for PHOs. According to a large national study, physicians contributed an average of 26 percent of capital, with primary care physicians contributing 12 percent and specialists contributing 14 percent, while hospitals provided the balance of capitalization.[7]

In the current market, the ideal ratio for both financing and governance of a PHO is 50:50. One way to achieve this ratio is for the hospital to match physician contributions, but this method depends on physicians' making a substantial contribution at the outset and on the number of physician participants. Physician organizations with more than a hundred members are more likely to contribute a satisfactory total amount than organizations with only a few dozen members.

Another option for initial capitalization is for the hospital to fully fund the PHO but to post a line of credit for physicians that they would repay through revenues from managed care contracts. Physicians financially at risk would also have a stronger incentive to manage care in a cost-effective manner.[9] Contributing a proportionate investment in a PHO may be difficult for some physicians, because, in urban markets, they may feel overburdened by requests from multiple hospitals. Furthermore, some physicians may resist investing because of having lost money contributing to past managed care ventures.

Despite physicians' misgivings, these joint ventures are relatively inexpensive compared to developing their own managed care organization and represent the necessary first step to participating in managed care. For many small group practices and solo rural providers, a PHO is the only opportunity to participate in managed care, short of selling out to a managed care company.[9] The start-up cost of developing a PHO is typically between $100,000 and $250,000, with costs of up to $500,000 for some of the larger multi-institutional PHOs.[7] Most of the development costs involve legal and consulting fees that increase as the provider panel increases in size and as the multi-institutional structure gets more complex.

Organization Management Issues

Funding for Operations

Daily operations can be funded by withholds from revenues obtained from managed care contracts, typically 2-5 percent of revenues. The hospital will usually contribute more for operations, however, because it generates more revenues than physicians. National surveys from 1994 document that the typical operating budget for a PHO is in the $100,000-300,000 range, depending on the numbers of providers and enrollees. An AMA study in 1994 revealed that the two largest expenses are staff salaries and benefits for general administration, marketing to managed care intermediaries, contract negotiation, medical management, provider relations, legal counsel, and management information systems.[9]

A PHO can minimize these operating costs by using hospital staff for some functions. For example, a PHO could use a hospital staff member on a part-time basis, thus benefiting from the person's expertise without having to pay a full-time salary. However, to avoid any tax or fraud and abuse problems, the PHO must have a signed leasing agreement with the hospital that adequately reimburses the lessor for the administrative professional and support staff costs.[9]

Information Systems

A significant start-up expense for all entities is funding a management information system. The ideal information system performs financial analysis, utilization management (prior authorization, concurrent review/case management documentation, and utilization review), data collection, physician practice profiles, outcome measurement reports with comparison to national norms, and other clinical quality assurance support reports. PHOs can easily spend several hundred thousand dollars on information systems that perform these functions. Instead of incurring this expense, many PHOs opt to outsource these activities to managed care administrators who charge for their services with a per member per month fee. As the volume of patients increases, additional revenues can eventually support moving the information systems functions within the organization.

Some PHOs have been frustrated by outside information system management services because some are third-party administrators that are not equipped to handle capitated payments or utilization management and quality assurance data analysis.[9] Other PHOs prefer to have total control over access to credentialing, financial (revenue and cost), provider profile, and medical management information and are willing to incur the expense of additional hardware, software, and interfaces.

Contracting

PHOs can enter into a variety of contractual arrangements. The number of contracts can be as few as one to well over 30. The number of covered lives can be as few as 1,000 for new PHOs in rural settings to well over 100,000 for more mature PHOs. The type of contracts typically depend on the age of the PHO and its managed care market. PHOs in markets with minimal managed care activity usually develop discounted fee-for-service arrangements with payers. PHOs in heavily penetrated managed care markets typically have both discounted fee and capitated contracts, with rapid growth in risk-based contracts. Most PHO consultants advise new PHOs to begin with simple, discounted fee-for-service contracts and then to gradually adopt more risk-sharing capitated contracts. For the first contract, many PHOs prefer to start with the hospital employee population, gaining experience with a relatively familiar market before contracting with outside employers. Other desirable contracts are typically with large self-funded businesses and local health coalitions.

Physician hospital organizations that receive capitated payments reimburse their physicians on either a capitated or a discounted fee-for-service basis using RBRVS or other national standardized reimbursement schedules. Primary care physicians tend to be paid under both scenarios, while specialists are usually reimbursed on a discounted fee-for-service basis. Many PHOs use provider withholds to manage risk, They typically withhold 15-20 percent of all provider fees and return the fees to all providers if utilization targets are met.[10] Otherwise, the PHO keeps the withholds to cover health care costs that exceed the actuarially determined budget.

This distribution method is less satisfactory for physicians if they are part of a larger group, because the individual physician's impact on cost savings is difficult to determine and reward. When risk is distributed among smaller groups and subgroups, physicians are more likely to see how their practice patterns directly affect their income. The most ideal arrangement, not commonly practiced, is to provide individual physicians with direct information and incentives to provide cost-effective care while still distributing nonprovider-controlled risk caused by specific catastrophic patients over a larger provider group.

These partnership organizations vary in their authority to bind physicians to joint venture contracts. Some physicians have granted PHOs the power to enter into contracts with payers as long as certain conditions are met, while other contracts allow providers the choice of "opting-out" of contracts within a set period if they are not satisfied with any of the agreement's terms. However, all physicians may legally contract separately with managed care health plans if they can obtain more acceptable terms.

A variety of payment methods for the hospital portion of PHO services is possible, with the most common method being DRG or per diem. Per diem payments consist of a fixed amount per day, regardless of the amount of resources used. Hospitals can make these payments profitable if they keep their costs below the payment rate. As PHO management expertise matures, they shift from a per diem rate to the higher risk method of a fixed per member per month payment. With proper medical management procedures and monitoring of resource utilization, hospitals can make inpatient care, or a lack thereof, a profitable venture.

Sometimes, an individual PHO or a network of PHOs will develop a state-licensed managed care financial intermediary as a means of becoming more competitive in the market. Hindrances to this development are the high cost of collateral associated with the assumption of risk, lack of expertise in marketing and member services, inexperience in third-party administrative activities, and negative impact on established relationships with insurance companies and other managed care health plans.[11]

Committees

Committees serve a valuable role in the PHO's development and ongoing operations. Many PHO responsibilities require analysis and decision making that is best made by a group that has dedicated the time and focus to a particular task. While committees are key to deciding developmental issues for any PHO, they are even more important in smaller PHOs that cannot afford a full-time administrator. In this case, the committees assume some of the responsibilities that a part-time administrator cannot address, because of either time constraints or lack of expertise. Further, committees composed of providers are better suited to address issues related to credentialing, provider selection, utilization management, and quality assurance because of members' medical expertise. Decisions related to revenue distribution and risk assumption are easier for the PHO board to make if a committee has already examined the issues in detail and made recommendations that reflect general agreement. The most common committee structure for a PHO includes an administrative committee for contract negotiations, revenue distribution, and selection of providers and a medical management committee with subcommittees for credentialing, utilization management, and quality assurance.

As PHOs accept more risk-based managed care contracts, the provider selection and review process becomes more selective, using objective outcome measurement data. Physician practice patterns become more significant as the managed care organization struggles to narrow its panel of physicians to those who provide high-quality, evidence-based managed care and are most cost-effective in order to create a small enough panel to make contracts profitable for individual members. The annual provider review process involves monitoring of utilization data, patient satisfaction data, quality assurance data, continuing education efforts, malpractice suits, and cooperation with PHO rules. Physicians who are deficient in one or more of these areas are provided with peer counseling; mentoring education; and, as necessary, outplacement counseling.

The committee dedicated to contract negotiations, provider selection, and revenue distribution typically does not have any difficulty recruiting members because of the high interest level of all providers. The PHO board and administrator depend on this committee to work through politically sensitive issues and to make recommendations that reflect compromise and realistic recommendations. The committee must determine the total provider revenue percentage of the premium dollar and the distribution to each provider type. The typical committee uses a mixture of per diem, age/sex capitation, and a percentage of a national standard professional component schedule (i.e., RBRVS). Sometimes, committee physicians will try to negotiate higher rates through the PHO than they would otherwise adopt in individual contracts.

Often, in new organizations, the recommended fee schedules are set at high levels to generate broad support among physicians. However, market forces will usually prevail; these high rates will be unacceptable to payers, who will refuse to participate. In these situations, the maturing PHO is forced to reconsider its rationale for premium pricing and to select a fee scale for all provider services that reflects the market-determined regional rate. Physician members must accept the realities of managed care. To better understand the market, the committee should consider conducting interviews and focus group discussions with managed care intermediaries and large employers. This research will help the PHO determine if a market exists for its product and to identify payment and service issues that will make the PHO more attractive in the new health care environment.

The credentialing, utilization management, and quality assurance committees do primary source document verification and monitor inpatient and outpatient care. Because continuous quality improvement and concurrent review programs to monitor inpatient care already exist in many hospitals, the committees usually collaborate with these services instead of duplicating them. Monitoring quality on an outpatient basis and developing case management methods usually require more of a committee's time, because ambulatory standards, medical management measurement tools, and comprehensive case management programs must be developed locally to reflect community resources.

These committees are also charged with monitoring total resource utilization review, which is especially important if the PHO accepts capitated payments. In this case, individual physicians' practice patterns are monitored to determine the extent of resource utilization relative to the payment received and the complexity of case mix and to make comparisons with regional and national provider peer groups. Most PHOs contract with managed care intermediaries for utilization management functions as a way to minimize their costs and efforts. However, if the managed care organization wants to mature into a true risk-taking entity, it must develop and control its own information and medical management system. Only through direct access to utilization and quality management knowledge and information can it use objective outcome measures, such as the HEDIS data elements, to accept risk, select providers, assign medical privileges, and be profitable in the managed care capitated environment.

Legal Issues

The "Statements of Antitrust Enforcement Policy in Healthcare," which was published by the United States Department of Justice and the United States Federal Trade Commission in August 1996, was written in response to the health care industry's request for more guidance on antitrust law regarding business activities of provider joint ventures. The antitrust "safety zones" build on the basic principles and concerns of antitrust law and maintain the law's fundamental restrictions and requirements.[10]

The "Statements" include guidance on the development of "exclusive" and "nonexclusive" physician networks. To prevent antitrust scrutiny, exclusive PHOs should have no more than 20 percent, and nonexclusive PHOs no more than 30 percent, of physicians in each specialty for a given market area.[10] Markets should be defined as broadly as possible. For example, a market for pediatric and adolescent medical services can include pediatricians, family practitioners, general practitioners, and internists as providers. Broadly defined markets are also relevant for PHOs that are developed in one-hospital towns with small medical staffs. If the town is located near another town or metropolitan area, the PHO can demonstrate that the local community has a choice of other providers, thus countering charges of monopoly power.[11,12]

Antitrust compliance typically involves risk sharing and economic integration. However, providers who do not share financial risk can still comply with antitrust laws through the following "clinical integration" programs.

- Medical management of care that monitors utilization to achieve cost efficiencies and ensure high-quality care.
- Credentialing and provider selection programs that contribute to a network's efficiency.
- Investment in infrastructure, e.g., information systems, that enables the network to monitor operations and outcomes.[10]

The revised antitrust laws also clarify the network's messenger model role. In a messenger model, a third party collects data from participating providers on fee schedules that they would be willing to accept. Acting on providers' behalf, the messenger may be able to contract with payers at rates that are equal to or better than providers' fee schedules. However, the revised antitrust guidelines note that the messenger cannot negotiate pricing terms, nor can it share the accepted fee schedules with competing providers. The messenger must also share with providers all contracting offers that fall short of their fee schedules so that they may consider these offers independently. Of utmost concern to lawmakers is that the messenger model not "create or facilitate an agreement among competitors" on prices or related price terms. If the network steers clear of such an agreement, it should be able to participate in a more flexible and active messenger model. However, PHOs should always consult legal expertise before embarking on such endeavors to ensure that they are in compliance with updated antitrust laws and interpretations.[10]

Conclusion

Physician hospital joint ventures that have physician and administrative leadership, operational management experience, appropriate governance, participative management style, adequate capital, and medical management knowledge have the essential ingredients for success. Providers must be willing to share financial risks and provide health care services to managed care members with utilization management and quality assurance monitoring. In order for medical management to work effectively, providers must invest their most precious resource—their time—by actively participating on administrative and medical management committees and in operational activities. Physician-led quality assurance and utilization management efforts are crucial to an entity's success. PHOs and POs that are undercapitalized, have members that have not accepted the realities of managed care, and do not invest time in developing the management knowledge, skills, and abilities needed in the managed care environment are prone to failure.

Health care is transitioning into a more integrated industry that assumes and manages both clinical and financial risks. Business structures such as physician hospital organization and physician organizations are needed to take providers from an independent, resource-rich environment to one that is highly integrated and has limited resources. Partnership health organizations can bring physician and hospital providers into a more integrated future, but these entities must be proactive and not wait until there is a crisis in the local service market. In PHOs, providers learn how to risk contract, manage a limited amount of resources, and provide cost-effective and medically effective patient care. All of these skills will be essential for all type of providers' survival in the future. By any measure, health care is moving into a new age, and provider joint ventures are its first evolutionary stage.

References

1. "Is a PHO Right for You?" *Medical Network Strategy Report* 3(4):4, April 1994.
2. Fromberg, R. "Can PHOs Work? Success Strategies and Lessons of Three Generations." *Health System Leader* 1(7):4-17, Sept. 1994.
3. Droste, T. "Physician-Hospital Organizations: Low Level of Integration Helps Doctors Handle Managed Care Contracts." *Medical Network Strategy Report* 2(4):1-3, April 1993.
4. Peters, G. *Healthcare Integration: A Legal Manual for Constructing Integrated Organizations.* Washington, D.C.: National Health Lawyers Association, 1995.
5. Gorey, T. *Case Study Analysis of Physician Hospital Organizations.* Chicago, Ill.: American Medical Association, 1994.
6. *Ibid.*, p. 18.
7. Hudson, T. "The Growing Pains of PHOs." *Hospitals and Health Networks* 69(1):42-5, Jan. 1995.
8. Gorey, T., *op. cit.*, p. 2-46.
9. Engstrom, P. "Where the Rubber Meets the Road: PHO Capital, Governance, and the Feds." *Medical Network Strategy Report* 4(6):1-3, June 1995.
10. Johnson, B. "Converting New Antitrust Guidance into Action." *Medical Group Management Journal* 44(1)22-6, Jan./Feb. 1997.

11. Gorey, T., *op. cit.*, pp. 11-12.

12. Engstrom, P. "Avoiding Antitrust Snags Requires Forethought and Thorough Market Analysis." *Medical Network Strategy Report* 4(5):1-4, May 1995.

Bibliography

Duncan, J., and others. *Strategic Management of Health Care Organizations,* Second Edition. Cambridge, Mass.: Blackwell Publishers, 1995.

Harris, J. *Strategic Health Management: A Guide for Employers, Employees, and Policy Makers.* San Francisco, Calif.: Jossey-Bass Publishers, 1994.

Kongstvedt, P. *The Managed Care Handbook.* Gaithersburg, Md.: Aspen Publications, 1993.

Shortell, S. *Effective Hospital-Physician Relationships.* Chicago, Ill.: Health Administration Press, 1991.

Wirth, T., and Allcorn, S. *Creating New Hospital-Physicians Collaboration.* Chicago, Ill.: Health Administration Press, 1993.

Eileen Weis, MHA, is Vice President, Janus Healthcare Consultant, Inc., Denver, Colorado. Kimball Austin Miller, MD, MSHA is Adjunct Professor of Business Administration, Arizona State University, College of Business, Department of Health Administration and Policy, Tempe, Arizona, and Adjunct Associate Professor of Medicine, University of Oklahoma, College of Medicine, Department of Internal Medicine, Tulsa, Oklahoma.

Chapter 6

Management Service Organizations

by Jeffrey R. Hoffman

Increasingly, health care providers, hospitals, large insurers, and even Wall Street venture capitalists are implementing strategies that integrate the fragmented pieces of our health care delivery system. The objective of this integration is to organize the disparate parts of the health care delivery system so they may assume both medical and financial accountability for the patients they serve. Restated in today's terminology, this integration positions providers and hospitals to "go at risk" for the care that they provide. Reasonable in theory, maybe, but in actual implementation, this integration is an evolutionary process for all parties involved and can take many years to occur.

Across the country, the speed at which local health care marketplaces integrate depends on many factors, the most important of which include the overall cost of health care services and of health insurance premiums in relation to those in other areas of the country, the size and number of large employers with purchasing clout, and the aggressiveness of local managed care insurers. Purchasers of health care insurance—employers and governments—as well as managed care payers, are encouraging integration of providers at the local level.

At the health care provider (physician, psychologist, advanced practice nurse, clinical mental health counselor) level, the growing specter of managed care and provider integration is placing clinical care providers under tremendous pressures:

- Declining fee-for-service revenue (e.g., fee discounting).
- Increasing managed care revenues, with complex financial incentives based on medical practice patterns.
- Rising practice overhead expenses.
- Increasing amounts of time consumed in administrative activities rather than in treating patients.
- Declining ability to attract new primary care providers to smaller practice sites.
- Increasing need for financial resources to invest in practice productivity technology and in contracting networks.

All of these pressures are forcing health care professionals to change the way in which they practice medicine and operate the business aspects of their practices. Primary care physicians, in particular, are continuously bombarded with offers to buy their practices, to join complicated managed care contracting structures—e.g., PHOs (physician hospital organizations), IPAs (independent practice organizations), POs (physician organizations), PSNs (provider service networks), etc.—or to invest in entrepreneurial business ventures devised to integrate the component parts of the local health care delivery system. Although these ventures generally begin the integration process through managed care contracting and contract management activities, they rarely address the day-to-day operational issues faced by most health care providers. The fact today is that, while many primary care physicians and mental health professionals experience practice changes initiated by the increasing development of managed care reimbursement, many providers are still reluctant to make the necessary changes in the way they practice and operate their businesses.

The management service organization (MSO) is an integrating structure that is gaining popularity among health care providers, mainly because it can comprehensively address key practice issues, such as overhead expenses, managed care contracting, capital investment, and administrative practice management. The MSO can handle these issues and still maintain a high degree of individual professional autonomy.

The remaining portion of this chapter attempts to address the fundamental questions that health care providers ask when they are learning about MSOs and considering whether or not to participate in an MSO. The chapter attempts to answer the questions health care professionals should ask, as well as provide additional questions they should receive acceptable answers to before they participate in any MSO venture

What Is a Management Service Organization?

An MSO is a legal entity whose aim is to provide management and support services to clinical practices The overall purpose of these services is to improve practice efficiency and productivity, allowing the individual health care provider to spend more time treating patients and taking home a larger share of the revenue generated by patient care activities. MSOs will typically own tangible practice assets, such as facilities and equipment, and will employ the nonprofessional staff of the private medical practice. The MSO does not employ clinical care providers or own patient charts, which remain in the control of the participating provider. An MSO is primarily a managerial, administrative, and support organization; it is not a provider of patient care services. The MSO acts as an integrating entity by taking individual independent practices and providing centralized management services.

Health care providers participate in MSOs through contractual arrangements that can take many forms. In the simplest form, individual clinical practices can purchase selected practice management services from the MSO a la carte (e.g., group purchasing services, information technology linkages, etc.). The practices will pay fair market value for the services they use.

Increasingly, health care professionals are choosing more in-depth involvement with MSOs in order to achieve the greatest benefits. In these arrangements, the MSO will purchase practice assets (e.g., facility, equipment, and accounts receivable) from the provider and employ all nonprofessional staff of the practice. The clinician remains independent. The MSO will manage the facility and the staff for the provider for a predetermined fee, generally based on a percentage of collected revenues. Under this arrangement, the burden of practice management falls to the MSO, thus freeing the clinician to spend more time with patients. By controlling practice expenses and seeing a greater number of patients, providers have the ability to maintain or increase their incomes even as markets become increasingly managed.

MSOs offer primary and specialty care practices a variety of services, usually broken into several categories: practice management, finance, and contracting. The table below illustrates many of the services provided to participating health care providers through an MSO.

How Are MSOs Structured and Controlled?

MSOs are generally structured as separate legal entities providing practice management services. MSOs are most often structured and controlled in one of four ways.

- Hospital-sponsored MSO.
- Physician/hospital joint venture MSO.
- Investor-sponsored MSO.
- HMO-affiliated MSO.

Services Provided by Typical MSOs

Management	Managed Care	Finance
Human Resources	Contracting	Billings/Collections
Practice Staffing	Negotiation	Group Purchasing
Scheduling	Claims Management	Budgeting
Utilization Review	Marketing	Information Technology
Quality Assurance	Member Services	Insurance
Physician Recruiting	Education	
Office Staff Supervision	Fee Schedule Development	
Staff Training		
Management Systems		
Practice Start-up		
Medical Records Systems		

Hospital-sponsored MSOs are the most common and are developed and financed by a local hospital or health system. These MSOs can be either tax-exempt or taxable, depending on whether or not the MSO is a division of the hospital or a separate entity, as well as on the ultimate purpose of the service. Under this structure the hospital will control the MSO's governance structure. Most hospitals invite community providers to sit on the governing board, but the overall number of providers may be limited to protect the hospital from concerns regarding inurement. Figure 1, below, depicts the relationship between the health system and individual clinicians in this type of MSO.

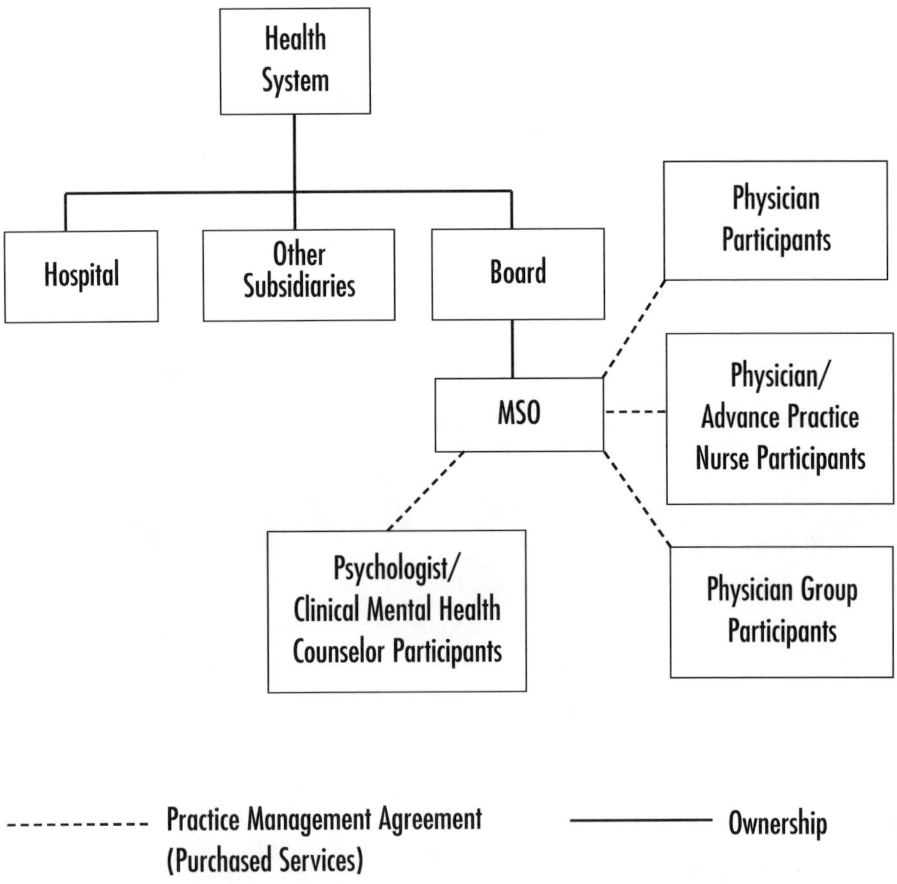

Figure 1. Structure of Health System-Sponsored HMO

In the physician/hospital joint venture MSO, a group of community providers and a hospital jointly invest in the development of a freestanding MSO. This entity would be taxable. Its governance structure would be developed on the basis of the levels of investment from the clinicians and the hospital. Figure 2, below, depicts the typical structure of a joint venture MSO. It would be created to provide practice management services and to allow both provider and hospital investors to earn dividends from a profitable MSO operation. Thus, investing clinicians could receive the productivity benefits of participating in an MSO and earn dividends from their MSO investment if the operation is profitable.

Figure 2. Structure of a Physician/Hospital Joint Venture MSO

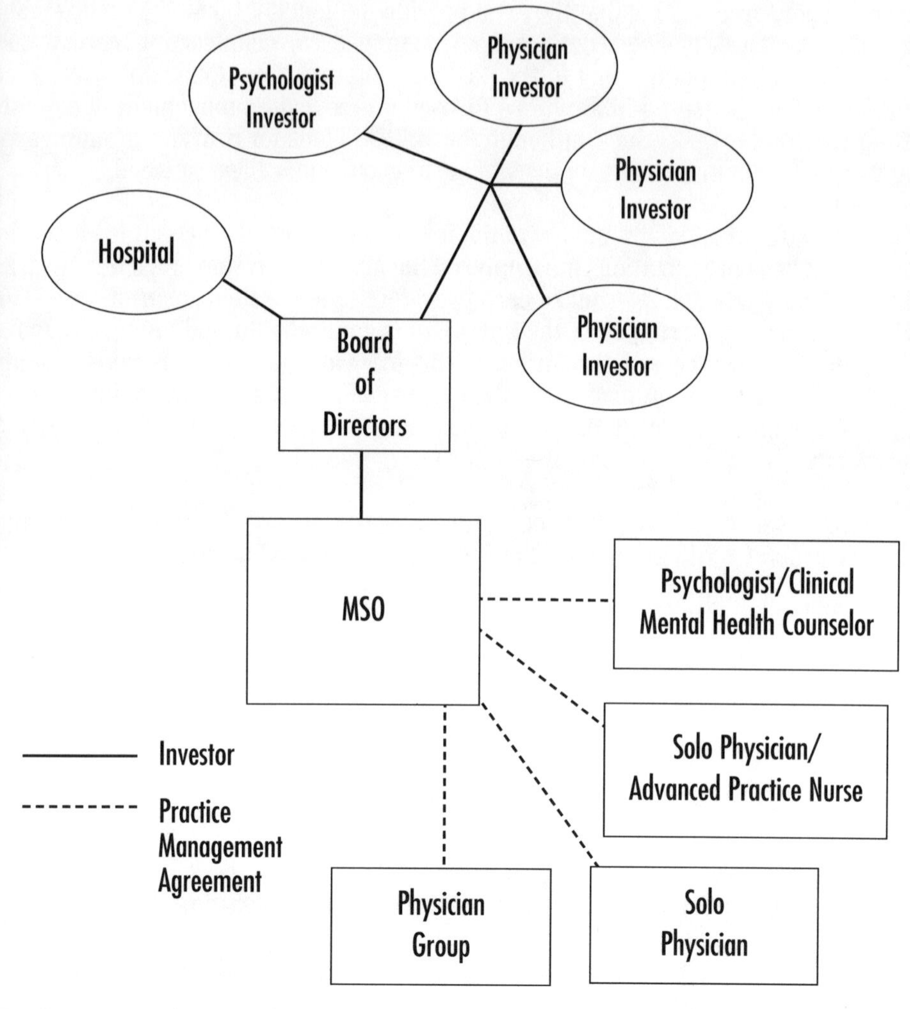

Freestanding MSOs can be created without a hospital partner A group of health care providers or private investors can be brought together to create the MSO operation. The main determinant is capital. If the MSO will be purchasing practice assets and developing information technology services, a significant amount of start-up capital will be required. The need for capital typically leads providers to include the local hospital or health system in the MSO.

Investor-sponsored MSOs are developed by large national companies (e.g., PhyCor, Caremark International, Coastal Physicians Group, etc.) or by independent venture capitalists who come into a local community and supply clinicians with the needed capital and management services. These MSOs are less inclined to provide only practice management services. Their main goal will be to organize networks of health care providers to contract with managed care insurers. These evolving provider networks will provide future value to the investor. The advantage of the investor-sponsored MSO is that they will provide immediate, turnkey practice management expertise, business development, managed care contracting, capital dollars, personnel, and marketing to the participating practices. Clinician governance in the investor-sponsored MSO will be focused on medical management of patients rather than on the operations, although the MSO will look for provider input regarding its practice management services to keep its customer base satisfied.

The HMO-affiliated MSO is similar to the investor-sponsored MSO but is owned by the HMO. These organizations have entered the arena to develop efficient networks of providers, particularly primary care providers to serve their insured base. The role for clinician governance of the operation is generally limited to medical management of the contracted patient base. This MSO alternative, while having some significant advantages in increasing the number of covered lives served by a practice, raises some uncomfortable issues regarding contract negotiation and clinician autonomy.

Overall, the success of any MSO venture, while certainly attributable to the organization's structure, will be more highly correlated to the following factors:

- Sufficient capitalization.
- Significant physician leadership.
- Experienced practice management.
- Service menu appropriate to the participating health care providers.
- Philosophy driven by high-quality patient care.

What Are the Advantages and Disadvantages of Participating in a Management Service Organization?

While there are multiple advantages and disadvantages in participating in MSOs, the majority revolve around practice productivity and efficiency, and around initiating the long-term evolution toward greater and greater health delivery system integration.

Advantages of MSOs include:

- The model is simple and easy to understand.
- Clinicians remain in control of their patients and revenue streams.
- Health care providers can have an equity interest in certain MSO structures.
- MSO development is often a preliminary step leading to primary care group practice develpment.
- MSOs, because of their flexibility, can meet the varied needs of a wide array of health care providers.
- Nonphysicians can invest, giving physicians and hospitals access to additional sources of capital.
- The cooperative arrangements that are developed may lead to further integrated relationships.
- Solo practitioners and small group practices can begin to take advantage of certain economies of scale previously available only to larger group practices.
- Health care providers are relieved of administrative management hassles and given additional time to see patients or use personally.

Disadvantages of MSOs include:

- To maintain health care provider autonomy, it is generally easy for providers to terminate the MSO relationship, thus weakening the MSO.
- MSOs require practice management expertise, which is difficult to come by.
- Remuneration in the hospital-sponsored or the physician/hospital joint venture model must be at fair market value.
- Fair market value limitations can put the hospital-sponsored model and the physician/hospital joint venture model at a disadvantage when they are competing with larger investor-sponsored MSOs.
- There are significant legal issues to be resolved when not-for-profit hospitals and clinicians attempt to develop an MSO joint venture.
- Significant amounts of capital will be required if the MSO is going to grow and develop systems that health care providers need but cannot acquire on their own.
- The MSO will constantly be changing to maintain its competitive advantage.

Why Should a Health Care Provider Consider Participating in a Management Service Organization?

Health care providers participate in MSOs for a variety of reasons. Clinicians in solo or small group practices will generally be attracted to MSOs because of their claims to lower the overhead of their existing practices. While practice expenses reductions are always good to consider, MSOs can offer significantly more. Many health care professionals underestimate the amount of time they invest in managing their own practices. By participating in an MSO, providers may be able to significantly enhance their personal life-style. In addition, the MSO can provide the dollars needed to bring to the participating practice the necessary information technology.

In summary, the principle reasons to consider joining a MSO include:

- Lower practice overhead expenses.
- Access to capital to acquire information systems or expand practice locations.
- Access to superior proactive business expertise.
- Ability to participate in a managed care provider network.

What Issues Should Be Considered Prior to Selecting an MSO?

Prior to participating in any MSO, health care providers need to analyze the benefits and drawbacks of participation against several general criteria:

- Up-front money (practice asset acquisition).
- Long-term income stability/viability.
- Clinician practice autonomy (i.e., control over medical decisions).
- Quality of care issues.
- Control over future strategic direction of the MSO.
- Information systems development expertise.
- Clinician participation in governance.
- The MSO's ability to supply needed business management expertise and capital to community practitioners.

To determine whether or not to participate in an MSO, health care providers must measure the MSOs in terms of all these criteria. Providers must also determine what priority they place on each of the criteria. To do this adequately, it can often be helpful for solo practitioners and provider groups to jointly use an independent facilitator, who can assist in structuring the discussion and a process by which a group of clinicians can reach a decision.

What Are the General Steps in the Process to Participate in an MSO?

As with any major financial transaction, there will be multiple steps for both parties involved. This allows health care providers significant opportunity to assess the transaction and to determine its potential benefit for their practices. While there are certain common steps to all MSO transactions, the uniqueness of each provider's situation and differing local health care marketplaces will lead to different responses. Yet transactions will have similar component parts.

First, think about and analyze some important questions:

- What do you want from your practice: money, personal freedom/lifestyle, autonomy, retirement, long-term practice options, etc.
- Do you understand managed care and its future importance in your local marketplace? MSOs are an opportunity to assist practices in developing managed care marketplaces.
- Do you require outside assistance to get what you need? This can be a difficult question for many health care providers to answer, because they are unsure of what they need to achieve their personal goals. The best advice that can be offered is: Make sure you are assessing the reality of your local marketplace. If you ignore real changes that are probably occurring, you will likely make the wrong decision.
- Do you want to sell practice assets or only receive management support services?

After you have determined your interest and evaluated several MSOs, the following steps will need to be taken if you want to have the MSO provide managerial services and purchase tangible practice assets:

- The MSO will conduct an evaluation of your practice to determine the fair market value of practice assets and to determine how efficiently the practice has been managed. This important step will lead to a financial offer for the practice assets as well as an indication of how much additional productivity the MSO can provide.
- The MSO and the health care provider will negotiate a purchase price and the financial arrangement to govern future practice management. The deal will most likely include a timed service contract for the health care professional. In other words, the provider will need to promise to remain in practice for a predetermined number of years under the negotiated arrangement.

As the MSO begins to manage the health care provider's practice, changes will occur, many of them determined in the negotiating phase of this process. Changes may include staffing, new contracts, new processes and systems, and investments in the facility. One thing is certain—the MSO, along with other integrating structures that health care professionals today are evaluating, will complicate the decision-making process. In dealing with these issues, providers should be assured of one thing, change is inevitable. It is occurring throughout the country. Following the status quo is rarely a successful strategy, and it is even less so today.

Jeffrey R. Hoffman is Manager of Strategy Services, Hamilton•KSA, San Francisco, California.

Chapter 7

Managed Care Contracting Models

by David A. Puffer and Kimball Austin Miller, MD, MSHA

The cost of health care in the United States has increased faster than the rest of the GNP. The *Fortune* 500 firms' expenditures for health benefits now equal 25 percent of profits. Much of the rapid increase in costs can be attributed to the cost of technology and to demographic changes, but this does not negate the need to manage health care costs. In response to this problem, most firms have become interested in alternatives to traditional indemnity plans in an effort to control their health benefit expenditures. Payers such as HMOs have grown rapidly as they attempt to offer an insurance product that limits health benefit cost increases.

The pressure to control costs is just as great at the government level. The commercial HMO products grew first, but the government is close behind. The federal government is encouraging HMOs to accept both Medicare and Medicaid patients. This process is accelerating and is generating new legislation. Cash grant Medicaid beneficiaries, such as Aid to Families with Dependent Children (AFDC), are being forced into HMO arrangements across the country. Enrollment in Medicaid risk programs is growing rapidly, and recent legislative initiatives attempt to accelerate the process. Every health care provider is being affected by these trends and must respond appropriately or risk being locked out of the market.

The term "managed care" is often used to describe any contracted or discounted medical products. A managed care contract, as used in this chapter, means a payer contracting process that requires providers to shoulder all or a portion of the financial risk for medical care and partake in utilization and quality review programs. HMOs typically meet this definition, as do some other payer organizations. As the variety of payer arrangements expands, it becomes more difficult to create clear classifications. However, if the agreement requires the provider to accept financial risk for medical services, the provider should expect additional obligations for coordinating care and group accountability for the cost of care.

Risk Contracting

Risk contracting with health care providers can take many forms. The manner in which health care professionals are organized (or not organized) determines the amount of risk borne by the provider and the means he or she has to control it. Five models of risk contracting are typical in the industry.

MODEL 1: Physicians Placed at Risk Individually by the Managed Care Payer (figure 1, page 103)

Managed care payers will often begin contracting directly with physicians, particularly when there is no physician organization (PO) set up to handle collective managed care contracting for a group of physicians. Primary care physicians are often paid on a capitated basis, while specialists are often paid on a fee-for-service basis. The managed care payer usually offers some sharing in hospital risk fund surpluses but rarely requires physicians to share in fund deficits. Because of the rise in POs, physician hospital organizations, and integrated health systems, this model is declining.

Model 2: IPA/Medical Group at Risk and Sharing in Hospital Risk Fund (figure 2, page 103)

Most managed care payers would rather contract with a PO that is structured to manage risk than with several independent physician offices. Medical groups are an obvious choice, but independent practice associations (IPAs) are also attractive operational formats for physician organizations. The typical IPA is a corporation formed for the purpose of contracting with payer organizations on behalf its contracted physicians. As illustrated in figure 2, the payer contracts with the PO to accept all risk for clinician and outpatient services and to share in the hospital risk fund surplus or deficit.

Model 3: IPA/Medical Group At Risk, Hospital Capitated (figure 3, page 104)

Managed care payers are interested in transferring all risk to provider organizations. The risk transfer can be accomplished by paying on a capitated basis not only the PO but the hospital as well. The hospital, in an effort to control its risk, usually offers the PO physicians surplus from its capitation fund. In mature managed care markets, hospitals prefer to be paid on a capitation basis by the managed care payer.

Model 4: IPA/Medical Group Capitated for All Services—Full Risk (figure 4, Page 104)

The full-risk contracting model holds the most risk and the most potential for financial reward for a PO. The full-risk agreement has the managed care payer giving the PO all of the medical and financial risk and all of the medical premium except for the managed care payer's administrative retention. The disadvantage is the significant amount of risk it picks up with this type of agreement. Most POs under a full-risk agreement negotiate a capitation agreement with a local hospital so that it can download some of the risk. Full-risk agreements are usually found in mature markets where POs have developed large patient enrollments and utilization management skills.

Model 5: Integrated Health System at Full Risk, IPA/Medical Group and Hospital Capitated (figure 5, page 105)

This full-risk contracting model has the managed care payer transferring all the medical and financial risk to the asset-integrated or virtually/contractually bound integrated health system. The managed care payer retains a portion of the premium for administrative activities, such as member services, employer relations,

Figure 1. Flow of Funds—Model 1

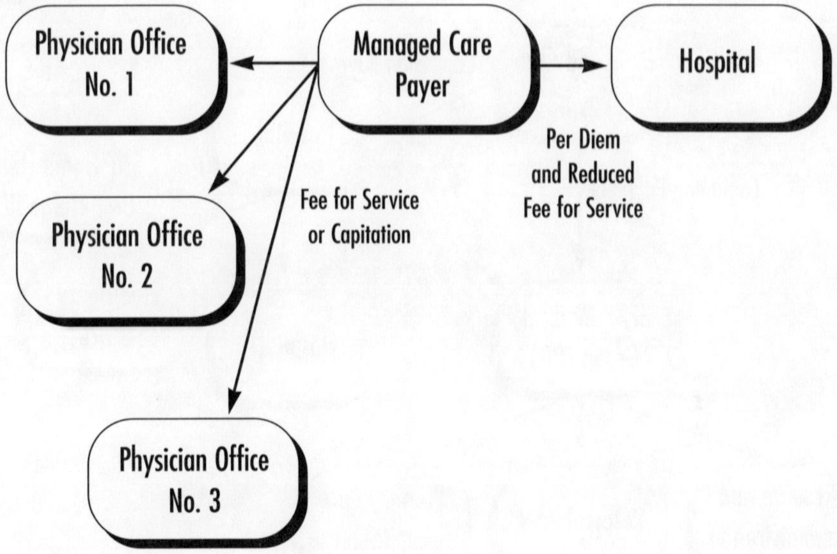

Figure 2. Flow of Funds—Model 2

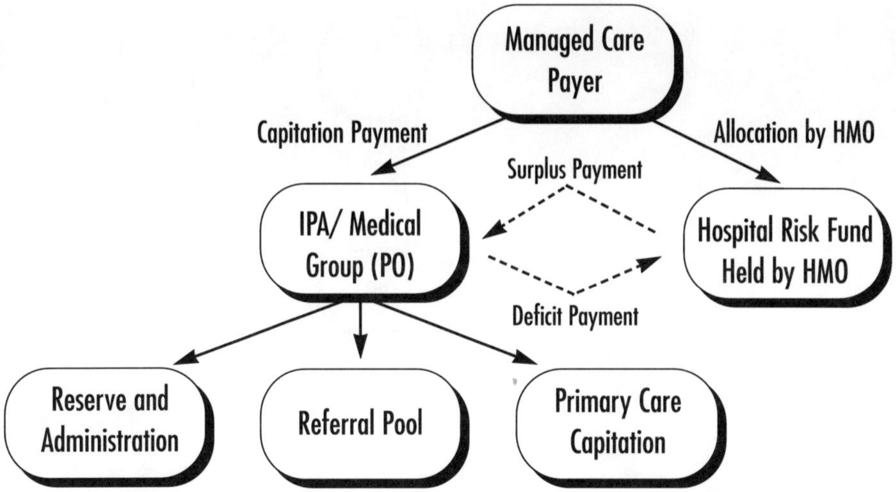

Figure 3. Flow of Funds—Model 3

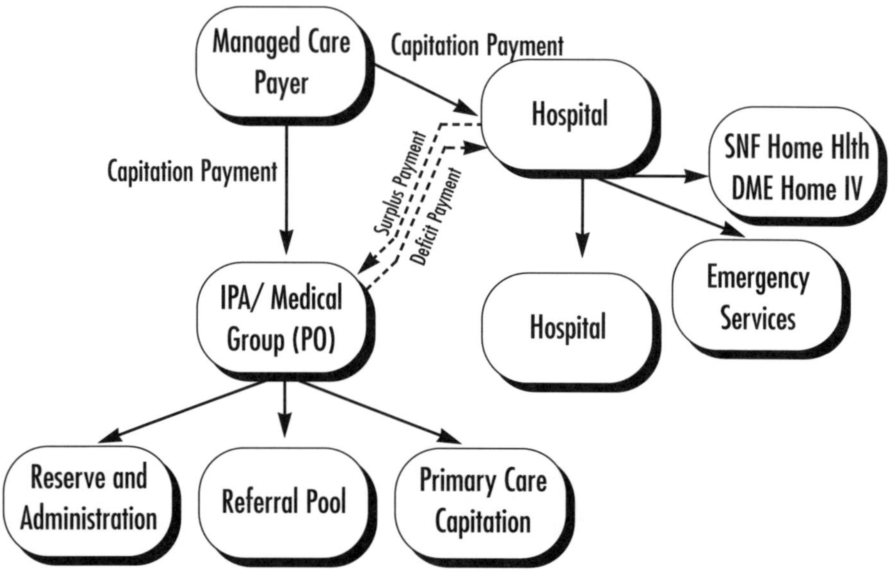

Figure 4. Flow of Funds—Model 4

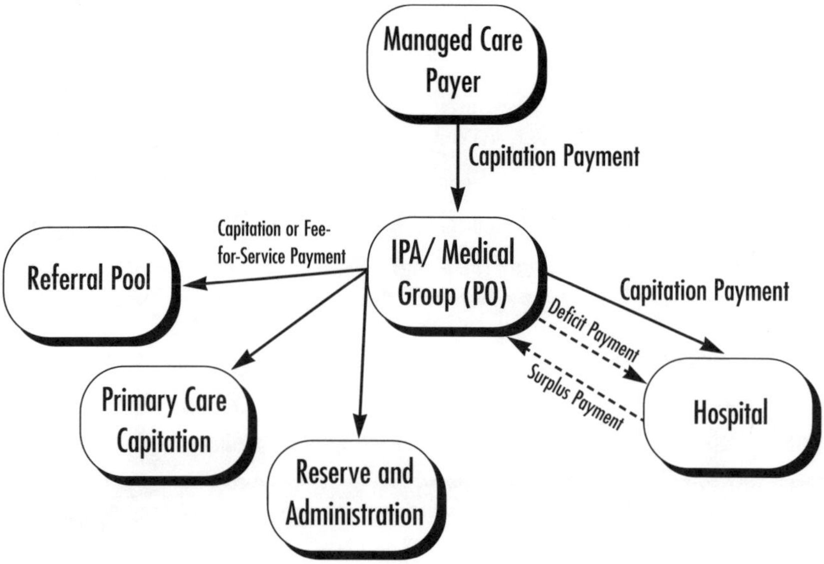

Figure 5. Flow of Funds—Model 5

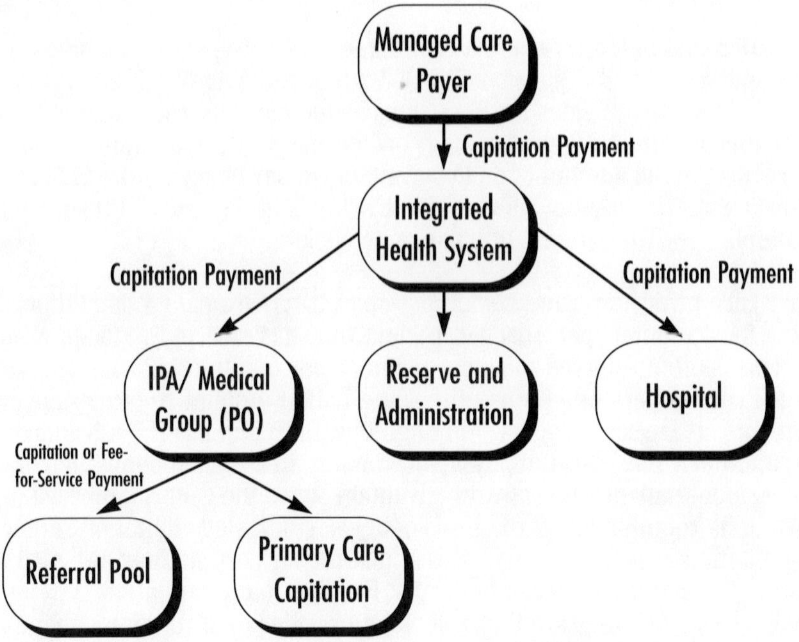

marketing, and stop-loss reinsurance. The integrated health system pays its PO and hospital partners on a capitated basis. The integrated organization must have effective utilization management, quality assurance programs, outcome measurement capabilities, and a fully operational information system. In this full-risk agreement, the integrated health system has the opportunity to retain all surpluses or distribute them to its organizational partners.

Provider Reimbursement

Health care provider reimbursement can take many forms. Often the payer or PO will pay on a fee-for-service basis, with a portion of the fee withheld pending the outcome of the risk funds. If the risk fund has a surplus, the provider gets the withhold back at the end of the contract year. If there is a deficit, the clinician may lose all or a portion of the withhold. Often, the return of a withhold fund is discretionary on the part of the holder, so that it can cover losses from other providers or to penalize a provider who has not been cooperative with the peer review process.

Many POs simply offer a lower fee-for-service reimbursement schedule and promise to pay out any surpluses in the health care provider fund to participating clinicians. This approach is conservative from the PO's perspective, because it allows the most flexibility. Because the typical PO has little or no capital reserves, the lower initial fee-for-service payment allows it to suffer adverse risk without having to reduce or delay payments to participants. The disadvantage to the provider is that he or she must wait until the end of the contract year to receive a surplus payout from the fund, assuming a surplus exists to be distributed.

A third approach to fee-for-service reimbursement is to pay on the basis of a floating multiplier. Often, the payer or PO will adopt the federal (HCFA) RBRVS or the McGraw-Hill Relative Values for Physicians as the basis for reimbursing physicians. The multiplier can be allowed to float on the basis of the amount of billings that exists relative to the amount of money available to pay claims. If the fund is five percent lower than the amount represented by claims, the payer or PO simply reduces the multiplier by five per cent to balance its books.

Primary care physicians, and sometimes specialists, are paid a capitation that is a monthly fixed amount per enrolled patient that has selected or been assigned to them. This is often referred to as per member per month (PMPM) payments. Some managed care payers or POs pay the same PMPM amount regardless of patients' copayments or age/sex category. Although this approach has the advantage of simplicity, it unfairly punishes the physician who has an assigned population of older or low copayment patients. It is always advantageous to the general internist and geriatrician to be reimbursed on the basis of age/sex-adjusted capitation rather than a fixed capitation because they will have older, higher cost patients assigned to them relative to other primary care physicians. Further, many capitation systems have a withhold or surplus program that will effect provider total reimbursement.

Capitation payments to clinicians are always contingent on retroactive adjustments to capitation based on retroactive enrollee additions or deletions. For example, if an enrollee who was reported on a health care providers capitation report is found to have terminated 90 days prior to the report, the provider's next capitation check will be reduced by an amount equal to three month's of capitation for the patient. Retroactive additions work in a similar manner. To account for both the revenue and the value of the services provided, most medical offices set capitated patients up under a special payer code. Each time a service is provided to a capitated patient, a charge is produced for this payer code. When the capitation is received, it is used to adjust the accumulated charges. If charges exceed capitation revenue, the excess is written off as an adjustment for capitation.

Any managed care participation agreement that requires the primary care provider to accept capitation should allow the provider the option of continuing on a fee-for-service basis until enrollment has reached an actuarially sound level for primary care services. Most POs will allow the primary care physician to be paid on a fee-for-service basis until at least 100 enrollees have selected him or her as their primary care physician.

The services for which the health care provider is at risk should be delineated at the CPT code level in the provider's participation agreement. If the services are not clearly defined, it is extremely difficult for the physician's office to determine which services are capitated and which are not. Also, if the services are not clearly defined, the PO or managed care payer can pay on an arbitrary basis. It is a good idea to exclude the cost of the most expensive immunizations from the capitation. The cost of live biologicals can be so great that there is a significant disincentive to give them. Immunizations are usually paid for outside of the capitation; they are often paid for on the basis of the local wholesale cost to physicians' offices, plus a modest dispensing fee.

Allocation of risk fund surpluses or deficits can be set on the basis of a rigid equation or at the discretion of the PO's governing board or of the administration of the managed care health plan. Because this is another form of reimbursement, often equaling 15-20 percent of total payments, it is important that the contracting health care provider have a full understanding of how funds will be distributed. If the payer or PO uses an equation, the physician must receive periodic reports on his or her performance. If the distribution is to be based on a subjective process, it is important that the contracting clinician understand the criteria being considered by the board. Therefore, in order to prosper in the at-risk relationship with health plans and provider organizations, all types of health care providers (physicians, psychologists, advanced practice nurses, clinical mental health counselors, and other direct care providers) must thoroughly understand the operational structure, policies, and procedures of the national, regional, or local contracting managed care entity.

Utilization Management

HMOs and other managed care health plans sell a benefit package that reduces or eliminates copayments while eliminating deductible payments by patients. The only person with an incentive to scrutinize the necessity for a service is the risk-taking entity. If the costs of medical services are not managed effectively, there will be insufficient funds to pay clinicians and hospitals. The very nature of the managed care agreement requires that medical services be provided on a cost-effective basis. The initial response of some health care providers to capitation payments is to adopt a strategy of denying referrals for care. Obviously, this approach will quickly lead to elevated costs resulting from underutilization of resources.

Most physician organizations and managed care health plans require prior authorization for some referrals. Elective referrals for outpatient specialty consults or treatment; diagnostic tests with a value greater than $200; and treatment by a nonphysician, such as a physical therapist, an occupational therapist, or a speech pathologist, all require prior authorization. Also, all elective admissions or outpatient surgery require prior authorization. Most organizations have policies allowing referral for services without prior authorization if the delay caused by the review process could jeopardize patient health. However, most organizations require concurrent notification of urgent referrals and review such referrals retrospectively. A current trend in utilization management is for the health care payer or PO to decrease its referral prior authorization activities and direct its operational emphasis and resources toward outcome measurement, provider profiling, and case management

Figure 6. Physician Organization Structure

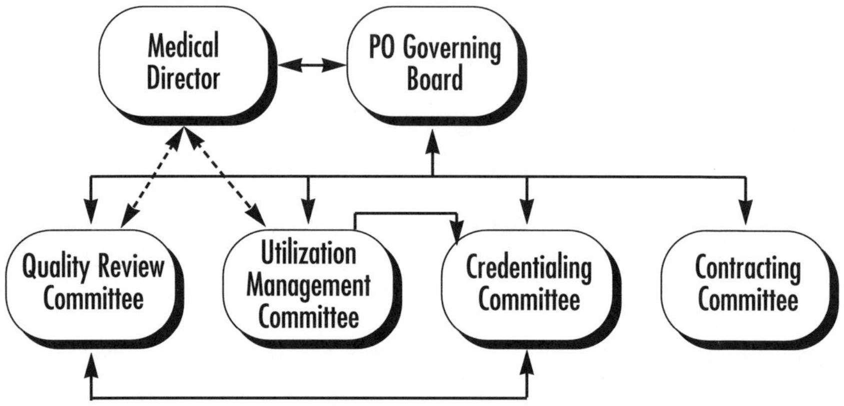

Most POs have a structure that holds the medical director and the utilization management committee (UMC) accountable for monitoring care. The medical director is charged by the board with setting policy and procedures for utilization management. The medical director typically chairs the UMC and the Quality Review Committee and reports committee recommendations to the board (figure 6). The UMC usually drafts all policies and procedures prior to making recommendations to the board. In addition, it reviews all elective referrals that represent difficult medical management problems or set precedence. It is up to the UMC to draft any prereferral clinical guidelines.

The UMC should be composed of a primary care majority, with specialists representing hospital-based physicians, surgical specialties, and obstetrics/gynecology. If Medicare or Medicaid populations are being managed, other specialties (such as orthopedics, ophthalmology, and cardiology) may be added. It is up to this group to set the strategy for managing risk for the PO. All health care providers participating in the PO should expect to receive guidance from the UMC so that they will know the basis of the review being performed on their referrals. Although the UMC reviews only exceptional referrals, it serves a very important function in this peer review-based process. All health care providers should be allowed to address the UMC if they disagree with the medical director's decision or with a policy issued by the UMC. Too many POs have started with the medical director as the sole decision maker, only to create a "benevolent dictator" approach to utilization control. The benevolent dictator approach almost always fails, because the responsibility for managing patient care is shifted from the care-giving clinician to the medical director.

Although the primary focus in controlling costs is through controlling patients' access to specialists, inpatient utilization is also important. The first line of defense in controlling hospital costs is controlling the decision to make an elective admission. The preauthorization process accomplishes this nicely. The second line of defense is to control the services ordered once a patient is admitted, the duration of the stay, and the transition from inpatient care back to outpatient care.

At a minimum, all risk-taking organizations should have a utilization management (UM) nurse on inpatient rounds, working with attending physicians to plan for the discharge of patients. When the UM nurse disagrees with the decisions of attending physicians, the PO's medical director will be notified so that he or she can consult with the attending physician. All health care utilization decisions must be made using objective clinical information, evidence-based outcome measures, and national and regional best practice clinical care guidelines. Furthermore, all clinical care decision disagreements must be reviewed by provider-staffed utilization management and quality review committees.

A second approach to utilization of resources management is to hire or contract with an intensivist to manage inpatient care. The intensivist, often a pulmonologist, rounds on all patients in the hospital for the PO. The intensivist may be made responsible for managing the care of all nonsurgical patients or may be empowered only to review charts and advise attending physicians.

Some organizations have delegated management of inpatient care to contracted groups of internal medicine and pediatric specialists who function as the sole managers of all urgent admissions and of all nonsurgical inpatient care. Under this arrangement, any PO physician who wishes to make an urgent admission would do so through this specialist. The inpatient specialists coordinate all specialty consults of patients until discharge. This approach has proved to be very successful when a medical group with a constructive attitude and strong clinical skills can be found. However, this strategy is usually used in markets where there is heavy HMO penetration and where health care providers are accustomed to the shared management of patients.

Quality Review

Each PO is contractually required to run its own quality review process. The multidisciplinary quality review committee (QRC) reports to the PO board and is responsible for reviewing all patient and health care provider complaints about quality of care and for conducting its own quality review studies. In addition to reviewing complaints and readmissions, the committee sets charting, acute illness, chronic disease, and health promotion care standards. The health care standards used by the QRC are peer developed using regional and national evidence-based medical care data.

As part of its oversight activities, the QRC may be asked to monitor patient access to care by conducting studies to determine waiting times for urgent care, minor acute illness, and periodic examination visits. The QRC conducts its business in a confidential process very similar to that used by hospital medical staffs and reports its findings to the board.

Provider Services Agreement

Each health care provider must sign a provider services agreement with the PO. This agreement governs all activities between the clinician's office and the PO. The agreement may have a 6- or 12-month term, with an automatic renewal. Some agreements do not have an automatic renewal and require the board to extend the agreement. To prevent contract problems, the service agreement should have specific definitions of such terms as medically necessary, emergency, primary care, urgent care, covered services, plan indemnification, and post-termination care. All agreements have provisions for termination without cause by either party after written notice is given. There will also be a bilateral provision for termination with cause. To avoid conflicts that could lead to termination of a contract, it is useful to have "cure" language in the agreement so that both parties can work together to resolve the difficulties.

The provider services agreement should contain compensation provisions. Although most contracts allow the PO board to revise compensation at its discretion, it is important to define the reimbursement basis in the agreement. Additional compensation provision may be contained in the PO's policy and procedures. Because these procedures are usually referenced and made a part of the provider services agreement, it is important that a health care provider read the policy and procedures prior to signing of the agreement. Along with compensation provisions, there will be financial sanctions for not cooperating with the PO. Providers should read these sections carefully and ascertain whether references are also made to them in the policy and procedures.

The health care provider's office will be held responsible for performing several clerical functions. Patient benefit eligibility verification, completion of referral forms, and submission of encounter information in a HCFA 1500 format are usually required. Furthermore, state agencies and business health coalitions regularly request health promotion, specific disease screening, and disease case management statistical data that will require medical practice/hospital staff time and effort.

Conclusions

Primary care and specialty care providers must participate in managed care contracting so that they can maintain practices. It is imperative that the health care provider read the participation agreement carefully and fully understand all aspects of this binding contract. Because the medical director and the UM staff will be reviewing all referrals, it is important that the clinician become familiar with their utilization and quality review approaches. This can be done by meeting with the medical director, by attending all PO managed care meetings, and by sitting in on UMC meetings. It is particularly beneficial if the health care professional can be assigned to the UMC for some time. The understanding of its process, plus the personal relationships that are developed in the process, can prove invaluable.

As was stated earlier in this chapter, health care providers should not enter into capitation agreements that subject them to adverse selection or insufficient compensation. Capitation payments must be age/gender-adjusted for an assigned population. Some POs will set expenditure limits (called a stop-loss) on the level of care per patient per year for defined conditions. Although the health care provider cannot avoid all adverse risk, it is best to be well informed of the PO's operations and to understand how to work through medical management problems with the UMC. A clinically strong practice that is open and cooperative with the UM and QR processes is likely to be given the benefit of the doubt.

Recent demographic health benefit studies are reporting the rapid shift of employed and public sector consumers of health care services into managed care health plans. With this swift decline in the indemnity fee-for-service patient population, all health care providers must quickly learn the operational structure, reimbursement design, medical management policies, and implementation procedures of the various managed care organizations and health plans with which they will have to interact. By moving up the learning curve, they will understand the new rules of the current health care delivery environment and not only survive but thrive in the evolving managed care world.

Bibliography

Kongstvedt, P. *The Managed Care Handbook*, Third Edition. Gaithersburg, Md.: Aspen Publications, 1996.

KPMG Compensation and Benefits Practice: Health Benefits in 1996. KPMG Peat Marwick, 1996.

Managing Managed Care in the Medical Practice. Chicago, Ill.: American Medical Association, 1995.

Roberts, M. *Your Money or Your Life: The Health Care Crisis Explained.* New York, N.Y.: Doubleday, 1993.

David A. Puffer is President, Pacific Managed Care Consultants, Inc. Laguna Beach, California. Kimball Austin Miller, MD, MSHA, is Adjunct Professor of Business Administration, Arizona State University, College of Business, Department of Health Administration and Policy, Tempe, Arizona, and Adjunct Associate Professor of Medicine, University of Oklahoma, College of Medicine, Department of Internal Medicine, Tulsa, Oklahoma.

Chapter 8

Vertically Asset Integrated Health Care Systems

by Thomas L. Kelly

Introduction

Business and economic historians will view the 1990s as an era of consolidation and rationalization for health care. (Rationalization is the restructuring of a business organization to reduce duplication of services, facilities, or support activities. It generally involves closure or conversion of facilities and reductions in numbers of employees.) During the 1990s, this rapidly expanding segment of the economy ran full force into market realities—changing technology, overcapacity, frustrated purchasers, and runaway inflation in health costs combined to remove the hot air from the health care balloon.

The integrated health care system (IHCS) was born as health care providers recognized and responded to the need for reduction in high-cost technologies; shift of care to noninstitutional settings; and long-neglected need for improved distribution of retail health care (i.e., primary physician care, physician extenders, physician assistants, and advanced practice nurses), home care, and related services provided in or near the home.

Since the early 1970s, there had been ample evidence of fundamental change in the health care sector. Building on the models created by Kaiser-Permanente and Group Health Cooperative in the 1950s, HMOs and PPOs, carve-out companies, utilization review organizations, and similar businesses expanded energetically in virtually every major market. These companies served as rationalizers of an overbuilt and undisciplined market. As they grew as an ever higher percentage of the commercial health care business, the flaws became evident in a model for health care delivery that was wasteful, of inconsistent quality, biased to expensive interventions, and all too often guilty of price gouging. For the most part, hospitals and physicians ignored the impact of the rationalizers, hoping and trusting that the comfortable health care guild of the 1960s and 1970s would be protected and preserved.

Consolidation and integration of health care financing and distribution activities are quite similar to attempts at vertical integration in other maturing industries. However, the capacity of integrated health care systems to develop or acquire the new skills needed for success in a vertically integrated business (e.g., insurance marketing and underwriting and medical group management) has not yet been conclusively demonstrated. Even more important, it is not yet clear that managers with an institutional (and often regulatory) mindset can adjust to the challenges of a rapidly changing market.

Key Elements of a Vertically Integrated Health Care System

The vertically integrated system is an organization that blends types of businesses that have been historically independent of one another. Its principal components—insurance, physician practice, and hospitals—are different types of businesses, requiring different kinds of expertise and management structure.

A vertically integrated health care system represents consolidation of the following activities:

Health insurance. The integrated system is committed to direct contracting with its customers, including private businesses and governments (both for government employees and for the beneficiaries of Medicaid, Medicare, or other tax-supported programs). In many states, the integrated health system must obtain either an insurance or a health maintenance organization license in order to bear risk

Regional hospital network. The integrated system needs to provide accessible inpatient and outpatient services throughout the region in which employees or beneficiaries reside.

Subspecialty clusters. As changes in health care technology have shifted significant amounts of medical care out of the hospital and into office-based settings, integrated systems have developed medical malls or clusters that provide a wide variety of subspecialty consultation, imaging and other diagnostic services, and often ambulatory surgery.

Primary care sites. An integrated system generally requires four or five times as many primary care sites as subspecialty clusters or hospitals to meet customer expectations of convenient primary care. Because most primary care medicine has been provided in solo or small group practices, the integrated system often needs to consolidate many small practices into larger practice sites in order to realize economies of scale and to ensure consistent service and clinical quality.

Retail medicine. Integrated systems must also give customers easy access to home care, physical and occupational therapy, counseling, dental and eye care, and pharmacy services. Often, these services are viewed as less essential to an integrated system's functioning and are offered through contracts or affiliations with independent organizations.

Many vertically integrated systems lack one or more of the activities described above, either as a result of specific market conditions that limit a system's span of consolidation, of partnering or vendor relationships with other companies that provide one or more of these services, or of being in the early stages of evolving into an integrated system.

Designing and Building a Vertically Integrated Health Care System

The design and development of a vertically integrated health care system generally requires assembling the various components described above. While several of the components may have been previously developed, almost always one or more significant components are not in place.

Key steps in the design include:

Creating a services model. The first step in the development of an integrated system is a detailed analysis of customer service requirements. Customer types—small and large private employers, union-sponsored benefit plans, government employers, and government-funded programs—must be separately analyzed, and a services map must be created to define the geographic boundaries of the market and the communities within the region that demand service access.

The service model should result in an inventory of needed services (both type and capacity), with a tentative matching of service needs to existing providers and an assessment of the likelihood that the needed capacity can be acquired or developed. Employers and union-sponsored benefit programs present the greatest challenge. Employees and their families covered by these programs often live at substantial distances from their employers and are often dispersed across a large geographic area. For example, in St. Louis, an employee of a downtown bank may live in Belleville, Illinois, or Wentzville, Missouri, which are separated by a distance of 75 miles.

Sequencing the integration. Once the service area is defined and an assessment of the needed services is completed, a health care provider or system wanting to develop into a integrated system must prioritize its integration activities. Most organizations find it difficult, if not impossible, to manage several merger negotiations at the same time. Even more difficult is the process of restructuring the organization to effectively manage the merged business.

A sequencing plan should prioritize acquisitions or mergers that will provide the best competitive advantage in the marketplace. For example, merger with another hospital that serves a separate service area in the same market and has a distinctive market franchise (i.e., is the clear provider of preference in that service area) would generally have a high priority. Similarly, an established medical group practice (either multispecialty or primary care) in a market without practices of similar size, managed care experience, or service and clinical quality would also be a priority merger or acquisition target. Hospitals with overlapping service areas or mixed reputations, small or dysfunctional groups, and ancillary providers (e.g., laboratories or home care companies) without substantial independent market strength would likely have a very low priority. The time needed to develop an integrated system provides an opportunity for aggressive competitor responses.

Establishing the core distribution system. Once the services model and the sequencing plan are developed, the most common next step is the establishment of the core distribution system. The core system is generally created through acquisition, merger, or affiliation of a series of hospitals. The principal objectives in forming the core system are to meet the geographic needs for institutional care (as defined in the core services model) and to provide a platform for acquisition and integration of physician practices in each key geographic market area.

Following establishment of the core distribution system, integrated systems often stagnate. The consolidated market share of the merged or affiliated hospitals will generally increase bargaining power and may cause the system to view integration as principally a defensive strategy. The merged hospitals may be able to prevent contracting with more attractive facilities unless a payer agrees also to contract with less attractive facilities or locations. With better ability to protect pricing and access to business, merged or affiliated hospitals may lose interest in completing the integration process.

Once a merged hospital group is created, three principal challenges remain—to acquire the ability to sell its services directly to the market, to rationalize its services, and to develop a companion physician services distribution system. These activities often take place in parallel.

Acquiring insurance capabilities. The health insurance system in the United States has provided a durable and significant buffer between the providers of health care services (suppliers) and the purchasers of those services. Prior to consolidation of health care suppliers, the insurance system has served as integrator of those services, purchasing services from a wide variety of suppliers and bundling individual prices into a single premium charge to the employer. Rapidly changing technology, rapid dispersion of that technology, inconsistent pricing structures, and volatility of the aggregate cost of services created the need for sophisticated administrative services and the capacity to absorb the cost risk to the individual purchaser.

Radical fragmentation of health care supply—thousands of individually owned companies providing a subset of services and the guild structure of physician services—ensured that suppliers could not deal directly with health care purchasers.

The acquisition of management and insurance capabilities by integrated systems is a logical conclusion to the rationalization of an expensive, redundant system of marketing health care services. It makes little sense for the vertically integrated system's services to be marketed by dozens of insurers who, for the most part, have no significant distinguishing characteristics and who retain 15-25 percent of the health care premium for administrative costs and profits. The integrated system, often representing as much as 70 percent of premium costs to the employer, finds itself unable to influence product design or pricing to the purchaser.

Integrated systems can offer simpler and standardized service pricing and already have the quality assurance and utilization management processes in place to meet the demands by customers for increased accountability. Because all or most of the services needed by a customer can be provided within the vertically integrated health care system, the insurance risks of underwriting a health plan can be dramatically diminished.

Thus, acquisition of insurance capabilities is an essential step in the development of an integrated system. By displacing the insurance intermediary, the integrated system can reduce marketing costs and develop the kind of supplier/purchaser partnership that is appropriate to the cost and complexity of health services.

Physician consolidation and integration. Solo and small group practice is the dominant form of physician organization. Practices operate as independent business units, with physicians or their office managers directly responsible for establishing office hours and service expectations, setting prices, contracting with insurers or other payers, and billing and collecting.

During a period of continuing increase in demand and limited, if any, focus on prices or quality, the solo/small group practice thrived. Revenues were sufficient to offset the substantial administrative inefficiency of the solo/small group model, and physicians were able to dedicate substantial time to administrative details while still earning attractive incomes.

More aggressive purchasing by insurers and consolidation of physicians and hospitals into networks and integrated systems has placed the solo/small group practitioner at risk. Access to contracts with insurers is not guaranteed; the individual and small group practitioner has limited ability to negotiate the financial and other terms of those contracts. The vertically integrated health care system may provide a safe haven for physicians, giving them market power they could never achieve individually. At the same time, integration brings with it the threat of lost professional and personal autonomy.

The primary care physician or subspecialist desires an integrated system with a demonstrated understanding of physician practice and with a commitment to physician leadership and decision-making processes appropriate to an association of professionals. Often, the integrated system will promise but not be able to demonstrate this commitment.

The continuing expansion of managed care has introduced several dramatic pressures into the solo/small group model. Through competitive contracting, payers have reduced the scope of services provided by physician offices and exerted considerable pressure on service pricing. By entering into exclusive agreements for laboratory, radiology, infusion, and other services, payers have removed profitable ancillary revenues from physician office practices. At the same time, payers have realized substantial discounts (often as much as 40-50 percent in more competitive areas) from prices for professional services. Solo and small group practices lack the leverage and the expertise to offset the power of the payer in contract negotiations and the size to realize operating efficiencies.

Along with pricing pressure, payers have imposed stringent new processes to manage utilization of health care services. Detailed, complex guidelines for referral of patients for subspecialty care, diagnostic testing, admission to the hospital, and care subsequent to hospitalization have substantially increased the administrative work load of physicians, taking more time away from practice and compounding the reduction of practice incomes.

The most successful physician response to payer contracting pressures has been aggregation into groups and networks. By organizing large numbers of physicians into independent practice associations (IPAs), physician hospital organizations (PHOs), groups without walls, and integrated groups, physicians have increased their leverage with payers and have been better able to afford expert legal and consulting assistance in contract negotiation.

For the vertically integrated health care system, aggregation of physicians into network and group structures has provided the needed groundwork for consolidation of physician practices into the integrated system. Networks and groups, often formed with minimal capital, soon discover the need for substantial investment in facilities, information services, and skilled personnel and the need for risk capital to protect the network or group from underwriting losses on risk-based contracts.

Vertically integrated health care systems are a good source of capital, and they generally share important values with physicians. A long-term commitment to the community, a history of cooperation and mutual dependency with physicians, and an organizational structure that can be changed to promote physician participation in leadership make physician/hospital partnerships a powerful response to market pressures, with excellent long-term prospects.

Because the integrated system is seeking to protect and enhance an already substantial investment in the community, physician groups and networks offer real synergies and permit lower expectations of return on invested capital than banks, insurers, or physician management companies are likely to have.

Thus, a principal component of a vertically integrated health care system is an organization of primary care and specialty physicians sized to match its institutional capacity. While an integrated system would generally prefer to integrate only or principally through established, efficiently functioning multispecialty group practices, the market realities most often make this option unavailable. The vertically integrated system generally must build its integrated group through consolidation and rationalization of new, poorly functioning practices, IPA or PHO networks, and solo practices.

Service rationalization. The merger of several institutions (the core distribution system) generally results in substantial redundancy of individual health programs and activities. This redundancy is compounded by changes in health technology that are rapidly shifting services to ambulatory centers, physicians' offices, and patients' homes.

The vertically integrated health care system will frequently find itself with a dramatic surplus of hospital beds in a health care community plagued by overcapacity. With hospitalization rates and lengths of stay continuing to decline, even the integrated system that is well-positioned competitively must focus on cost reductions and improved efficiency of operation.

Service rationalization can take a variety of forms: closure or conversion of less attractive inpatient facilities; consolidation of clinical specialties (e.g., cardiovascular or orthopedic services) at one facility; consolidation of ancillary services (e.g., clinical laboratories, home care, infusion services, and the like) into a single, independent organization; and consolidation of administrative activities (including systems, accounting, human resources, marketing, planning, legal, and patient billing).Without rationalization, the vertically integrated health care system cannot produce the capital needed for physician consolidation and for acquisition of insurance functions and cannot achieve the economies demanded by its customers.

Governance Models for the Vertically Integrated Health Care System

To be successful, a vertically integrated health care system must retain or acquire experienced leadership in each line of business and blend that leadership at the parent company level to ensure that consolidated business plans and strategies reflect a sophisticated understanding of each line of business.

The physician component of the vertically integrated system presents the most significant challenges to the governance of an integrated system. While insurance and institutional health care businesses are accustomed to structured decision-making processes and executive leadership models, physicians are a blend of small business owners and entrepreneurs or are group participants accustomed to consensus-based decision-making at a board or shareholder level. Further, whether physicians are in solo/small group practices or larger medical groups, the most common models for decision making have involved physicians in most routine operating decisions (e.g., staff hiring, fringe benefit plans, supply or equipment purchases, price setting, and medical record formats). Thus, the physician comes to the vertically integrated system ill-prepared for a corporate governance and management model, and the insurance and institutional components come with little, if any, understanding (or appreciation) of physician consensus-style decision making.

As a result of these fundamental differences in approaches to governance and decision-making processes, the integrated system must devise a governance model that permits each line of business to operate effectively. At the same time, the governance organization must ensure that the parent company has the capacity to set common strategic and business goals and to allocate resources in a manner that obtains the active support of senior managers in each line of business.

Reasons for Success and Failure of Vertically Integrated Health Care Systems

A vertically integrated health care system is a dramatic adaptation to a changing market. With increased leverage with its customers and the ability to bypass insurers, the integrated system can substantially improve its performance. At the same time, a vertically integrated system is well positioned to systematically improve the effectiveness of health care delivery, because all health providers are assembled in a single organization with a shared definition of success. Of course, any combination of fundamentally different businesses brings with it a significant risk that executive leadership and the board may not have the capacity to lead and govern the new organization.

Operating inefficiency. By consolidating many independent entities—physician groups, hospitals, payers, ambulatory facilities, and the like—into a single, vertically integrated organization, the integrated system has the opportunity to realize substantial economies. By combining redundant programs and services and reducing overhead, the vertically integrated system can gain significant cost advantages over its fragmented competitors. At the same time, one of the most common reasons for integration—market power—leads all too often to its long-term demise. The larger, more powerful integrated system finds itself able to resist market pressures for efficiency and may be able to force the market to accept a more costly, lower quality product or service than a more competitive market may have tolerated.

Poor management skills. Integrated systems have the capacity and complexity needed to attract and retain leaders with top-quality skills. A vertically integrated system can and should have marketing, underwriting, physician management, financing, and other business management expertise not available to smaller organizations. Powerful business and professional leadership provides a substantial competitive advantage to the integrated system. Yet, all too often, hospital managers have dominated the senior management of integrated systems and have brought to their expanded responsibilities either an unwillingness or an incapacity to understand the impact of changing markets and technology or to appreciate the management needs of substantially different types of businesses.

Imperfect adherence to the service model. The success of any integrated system is a function of having the right combination of physicians, hospitals, and other organizations. When the aggregated organization yields competitive advantages in distribution, quality, public recognition, and so forth, the integrated system has substantially improved chances of success. Alternatively, many vertically integrated health care systems have been formed through the merger and consolidation of hospitals whose selection was based principally on friendships among key managers or common organizational types (e.g., nondenominational not-for-profit, for-profit, or religious-affiliated not-for-profit), without due regard for market needs or for the relative market strength of each organization. When integrated systems ignore fundamental needs, the resulting organization often poorly fits the market or has structural weakness that can damage its prospects for long-term success.

Poor timing or poor strategic fit with market. A successful integrated system strategy is more often pro-active (i.e., anticipating market changes) than reactive. An early starter in the integration process can often choose its member organizations more freely and has the time and opportunity to sell its strategic vision without the noise and confusion created by competition. The organization that is a late starter in the integration process is likely to find fewer attractive merger partners. Further, merging organizations, particularly physicians, are likely to extract a higher merger premium—for example, financial or governance protections—when the integrating organization does not appear to be a market leader. With less likelihood of long-term success and less ability to harm the merger partner competitively, the weaker integrating system must pay more to its merger partners. In adopting an integration strategy, an organization must objectively assess the likelihood of market success. Market leadership and service to all or most of the service area, with no dramatic weaknesses, are key elements for success.

Insufficient capital or planning. The merger and consolidation of well-capitalized, profitable, and well-managed organizations often involves substantial dislocation of senior management resources (both during and after the transaction). The vertically integrating organization must recognize and plan for these realities. Key constituencies—board members and senior leadership of all merging organizations—must understand and accept the complexity of the consolidation process and endorse the capital and personal investments needed to complete the plan if the venture is to succeed.

A poorly capitalized organization may not be able to afford the costs of rationalizing the consolidated businesses. If not properly anticipated and presented to key constituencies (boards of directors and rating agencies), merger-related losses can have a substantial adverse impact on continuing board support or may result in reduced access to capital. Lack of management attention to the continuing operating needs of the combining businesses may result in deterioration of business performance or of market reputation.

Summary and Conclusions

Large integrated health care systems involve horizontal integration of businesses and individuals providing health care services and vertical integration of service and financing activities in health care. The primary goal of integrated systems is increased market share during an era in which changing technology and increased sensitivity to health care costs have resulted in dramatic service overcapacity.

Horizontal integration aims to increase market leverage. The principal objectives of vertical integration are to improve access to the customer, reducing marketing and administrative costs and resulting in a more durable, long-term association.

The more substantial impediments to development of an integrated system include the design of a service model that is achievable and that will enhance the organization's market power. The vertically integrated system must serve all, or the majority, of a market's needs for health care services. It must achieve orderly and efficient integration of physician, hospital, and insurance functions and must create a governance model that permits effective management of diverse businesses with fundamentally different expectations about the structure of decision making. Perhaps as important, the vertically integrated system must be a timely response to changing conditions in the market, achieved at an affordable capital cost to the merging parties.

Before embarking on an integration strategy, any major provider or insurer or organization must answer the following key questions:

- Does the organization have the capacity and will to strengthen my organization through systematic consolidation and rationalization of regional provider and insurance functions?
- Are the constituent parts needed to form an integrated system available for merger/acquisition, or does the organization have the capability to invent those constituent parts?
- Is the organization ready to accept the loss of governance and senior leadership control that almost inevitably accompanies a business transformation of this magnitude?

Affirmative answers to these questions lead the regional provider or insurer to a vertically integrated strategy that, if successful, has demonstrated a superior ability to gain and hold profitable market share and to assist in rationalization of a fragmented business with inefficient deployment of capital.

In considering whether to sell or merge a clinical practice or health care facility as part of the formation of a vertically integrated health care system, a health care professional must answer a similar series of questions:

- Will the vertically integrated system survive and prosper?
- Will it achieve the increase in market strength it seeks?
- Does the leadership of the integrated system have the capacity and will to follow through?
- Does the vertically integrated system understand and value providers?
- Has the system put in place a governance and management model that will prove attractive to health care practitioners other than me?

- Does the system have the capital and the profitability to meet its current and future obligations?
- Will I like my profession and my place of work five years from now?

Affirmative answers should lead the health care professional to a careful evaluation of the opportunity to integrate. Any "no" is significant and may suggest that another route is preferable.

Thomas L. Kelly is President and CEO, Mercy Health Plans, St. Louis, Missouri.

Chapter 9

Vertically Integrated Health Care Systems

by Leonard D. Schaeffer and Dana E. McMurtry

Introduction

Market forces are rapidly reshaping the way in which health care is delivered and financed. Increasingly sophisticated purchasers—employers and government—require health plans to compete on factors other than just price: quality of care, customer service, broad geographical access, and choice of products, including point-of-service options and workers' compensation managed care products.

In addition to responding to market pressures, health plans must compete within the constraints of an increasingly restrictive regulatory environment. The demise of federal health care reform in 1994 did not dampen individual states' interest in addressing the problems of the uninsured. More and more states are adopting insurance reform laws to prevent the strategies traditionally used by indemnity carriers to compete for business—segmenting the market, increasing prices, and aggressive underwriting.

Health plans are responding to the fierce competition and the complex and uncertain regulatory environment by adopting new organizational forms that generate savings by aligning incentives to change provider behaviors and to provide high quality, cost-effective care. Health plans of the 21st Century will focus on integrated health care delivery approaches in which organizations and individuals focus on their respective competencies in order to manage care. Managing care—that is, coordinating care along a continuum of services—depends on the extent to which the organized system can integrate key support functions (financial management, information systems, marketing, etc.) and to which health care providers are economically linked and committed to the overall success of the system.[1] The form integration takes, however, may not be vertical, with all components belonging to one organization, but "virtual," with alliances and partnerships used to align interests to create even stronger bonds than ownership.

Market Transition to Managed Care

The emergence of managed care as the dominant mode of delivery presaged the more recent phenomenon of managed care organizations, insurers, and providers developing integrated delivery systems. Since the early 1980s, HMOs, which seek to meld insurance and health care delivery, have seriously challenged the dominance of commercial plans and the Blue Cross/Blue Shield system.

In bellwether states, such as California, the market is moving rapidly toward managed competition, in which managed care plans compete with one another and traditional fee-for-service plans are practically extinct. Before reaching managed competition, however, markets move through a number of stages in which all the players continually adapt in response to shifting power relationships (figure 1, below).[2] A decade or two ago, most markets were mainly fee-for-service, with less than 10 percent HMO penetration. The oversupply of hospital beds encouraged overuse of hospital care. These unstructured markets start to change as managed care entities emerge and employers begin encouraging workers to switch to managed care products. The prevalence of fee-for-service (FFS) plans inhibits the ability of HMOs and PPOs to get sizable discounts until their patient volume begins to grow.

Figure 1. Stages of Market Evolution

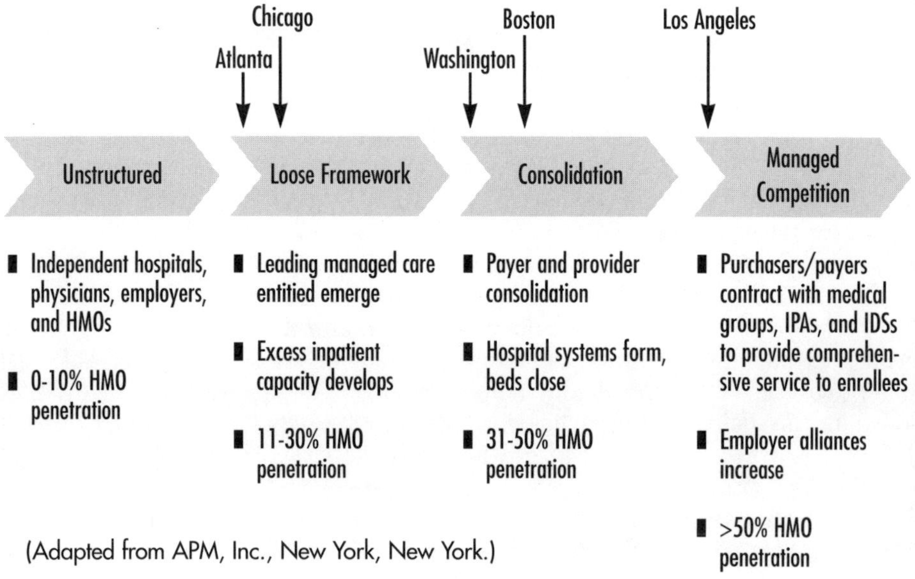

(Adapted from APM, Inc., New York, New York.)

Once these managed care entities gain market share, they capitalize on the oversupply of hospital beds and specialists and accelerate the elimination of inefficiency from the system. Health plans consolidate as a growth strategy and to spread administrative costs across a larger membership. Physician practices and hospitals also consolidate in order to win contracts with health plans by providing services at lowest cost.

Under managed competition, managed care plans compete for rural and remote areas and also for Medicaid and Medicare populations. The intense competition fosters even more payer and provider consolidation, in part, because of the need for coordinated delivery of care on a regional basis. It also fosters aggregation of purchasers into regional purchasing alliances to increase negotiating clout for lower cost products. In this buyer-driven market, integrated delivery systems develop to contract with payers, but some also try to integrate financing and delivery in ways resembling traditional HMOs. Ultimately, previous strategies based on exploiting excess capacity and the oversupply of specialists give way to new models of care as a means of controlling costs.

Approaches to Integration

The term integrated delivery system (IDS) is generally used to describe how provider delivery systems and/or insurance companies consolidate their respective roles and services to combine financing and delivery under one umbrella organization. There is certainly no single or succinct definition of an integrated health system. Instead, there has been some confusion, because there are a number of integration models competing in the market today.

Shortell conceptualizes four prototypes that are being tested in the marketplace.[3] The "integrators" in these models are led by hospitals, physician groups, physician/hospital organizations (PHOs), and insurance companies (figure 2, below).

Figure 2. Marketplace Testing Different Models[3]

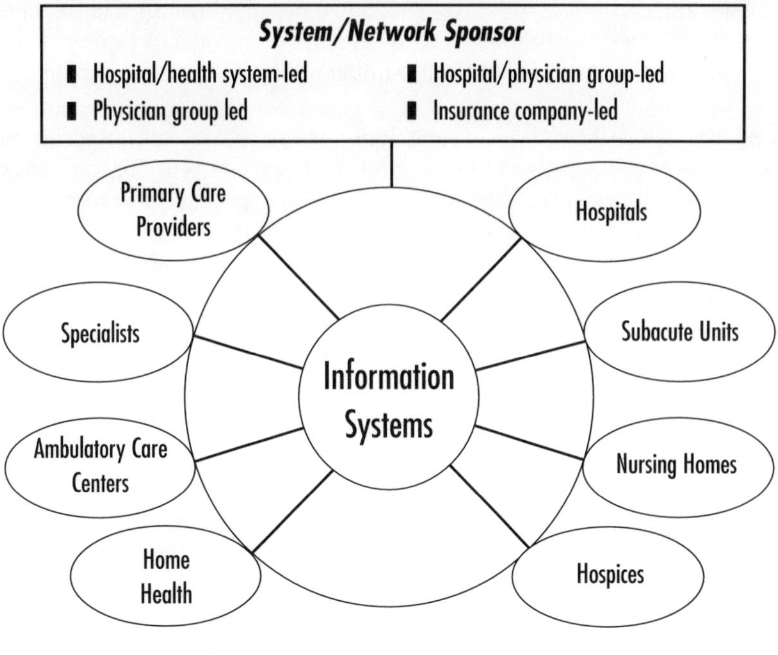

Payment mechanisms for these models range from fee for service to capitation. In addition, while some provider-initiated models incorporate the insurance function in order to directly contract with purchasers, many contract with HMOs or insurers to achieve the same coordination of financing and delivery.

At a minimum, integrated delivery systems include networks of health organizations that provide or arrange to provide a continuum of services to a defined population for which they are held clinically and fiscally accountable.[1,4] Currently, integrated delivery systems are accountable for cost-effective delivery of health services. As organized systems mature, that accountability will move beyond managing care to managing health as well, while still controlling per capita costs. Potentially, as the market consolidates to fewer health plans that also enroll Medicare and Medicaid beneficiaries, these plans may be expected to assume greater accountability for a community's health status.

Until recently, the concept of integrated delivery systems seemed to refer mainly to models that included vertically integrated systems, such as Kaiser Permanente. Now the concept has been broadened to include not only joint ownership, but systems linked together through contractual relationships, the basis of virtual integration. The three basic approaches to integration include.[1,4]

Full ownership. Given the prominence of Kaiser, this "bricks and mortar" model may be the best known. In the lexicon of integration, it can mean full vertical integration, in which the insurance, hospital, and physician components are owned and operated by a single corporate entity. However, it can also refer to horizontally linked entities that do not include the insurance component but focus on owning a segment of the delivery system, such as a hospital or physician practices, obtained through acquisition. Columbia/HCA and Mullikin are two prominent examples.

Joint venture. There are several variations on this model, although in each the jointly owned entity is jointly governed and profits/losses are shared. Advantages include not having to raise additional capital and creation of an equity relationship without the need to form a separate business. Models include partnering of an insurance company or HMO with a physician group or hospital to jointly own an HMO, PPO, or point-of-service (POS) plan; a delivery system; or a specific product. It also includes a narrower form of integrated delivery system, physician hospital organizations (PHOs), in which one or more hospitals link with attending physicians and/or other physician groups to seek managed care contracts, usually on a capitated basis. According to a 1995 survey,5 about a third of PHOs plan to seek licensure as health plans in order to directly contract with private and public purchasers.

Contractual relationships. This model is characterized by agreement to share risk. Partners are linked only through contractual arrangements and no separate legal entity is created. Varying degrees of risk are assumed through payment arrangements that include capitation, partial capitation, and discounted fees. Management services organizations (MSOs) would also be included, although they may be joint ventures as well. MSOs provide administrative and management functions to health care provider groups to relieve them of business responsibilities. In some cases, the MSO owns the provider groups' assets.

Genesis of the Term "Virtual Integration"

The contractual approach to integration in order to improve system performance and create value for customers has been dubbed "virtual integration," a term borrowed from Ernst & Young's Stephen Burrill.[5] Burrill used the term to describe the strategy used by biotechnology firms to "increase the number and variety of external relationships and operations without increasing staff or building facilities."[6] Biotech companies have discovered that virtual integration allows them to bring expertise in-house or to "cherry pick" contracted services.[7] In addition, they have learned that it is not necessary to physically control all of the value chain nor is it possible for one company to master every facet of their business. Rather, it is more important to be able to "extend strengths and access the strengths of others."[8]

In his seminal article, "The Illusive Logic of Integration," health futurist Jeff Goldsmith questions whether systems can, in fact, be *too* integrated.[6] In comparing the performance of Kaiser to other less integrated systems, such as Pacificare, HealthNet, and WellPoint, Goldsmith concludes that the "bricks and mortar" approach is less able to compete with systems whose principal assets are information systems and cash. According to Goldsmith, two key elements hold virtually integrated systems together and make them profitable:

- The operating system—i.e., the framework of agreements and protocols that governs how patients are cared for, as well as the information systems that monitor the flow of care.
- The framework of incentives that governs how physicians and hospitals are paid.

Although virtual integration may be advantageous for the consumer, a number of advantages also accrue to the partnering organizations. For the smaller entity, the partnership may bring access to capital, new markets, technology, established distribution channels, and greater credibility that can be used to secure financing and attract customers. For the larger firm, the alliance is often tactical, because its growth strategy does not have to rely on expensive, time-consuming internal development. Instead, the firm gains access to a broad range of products and technologies without exposure to the risks and costs of development. In addition, the firm identifies opportunities for acquisition, but has the time to assess the uncertainty and probability of success.[9] The larger firm also benefits from the "entrepreneurial" spirit that virtual integration fosters through contracting arrangements.

Virtual integration is based on the belief that aligning interests can create even stronger bonds than can ownership or employer/employee relationships. Vertically integrated systems that seek to acquire medical practices and employ physicians effectively eliminate the physician's risk. Solo practitioners and even medical groups lose the "entrepreneurial" incentive to scrutinize their clinical practices to ensure quality and to manage their own costs. Unable to successfully self-regulate, the umbrella organization finds it necessary to adopt a strategy of adversarial enforcement of standards relating to treatment and quality. Otherwise, all investments in systems and protocol development to reduce practice variation are wasted at the point of service. In contrast, contractual relationships in virtually integrated systems continually pressure providers to focus on their clinical skills and resource use in order to win and retain contracts.

Theory versus Practice

Tightly organized structures—i.e., fully owned, vertically integrated systems—are unlikely to win the Darwinian struggle and emerge as the delivery system of the future in most markets. Despite their theoretical elegance, such systems have not exhibited the economies of scale, coordination of care, and better health outcomes necessary to outcompete contractually linked, virtually integrated systems. Vertically integrated systems do not automatically lead to lower costs for a number of reasons, ranging from problems inherent in their structure and management to difficulties of merging different professional cultures (figure 3, below).

Organized health systems that rely heavily on ownership of facilities and exclusive provider relationships tend to foster bureaucracies that frustrate patients and clinicians. Managerial hierarchies that must include representatives from all the components complicate decision making, which must be swift to keep up with changing markets. Vertically integrated medical systems simply cannot adapt fast enough to accommodate changing preferences among consumers.

Figure 3. Alternative Approaches to Integration

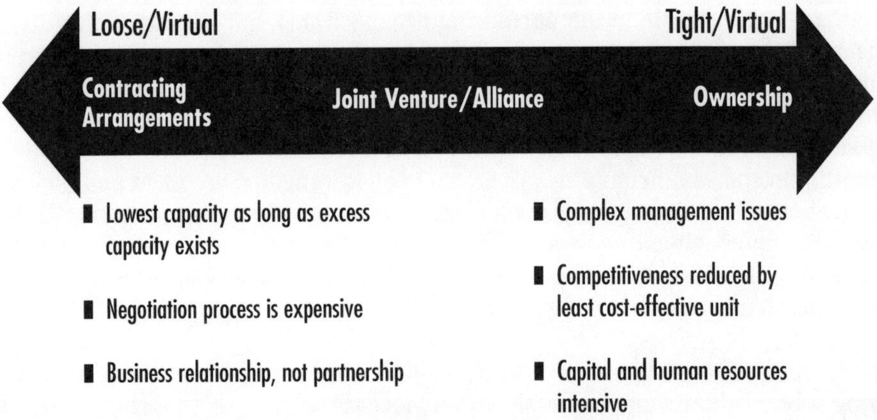

Adapted from Edward O'Neil, Presentation to Blue Cross/Blue Shield Association, 1995.

In tighter structures, the least cost-effective unit can threaten the overall competitiveness of the system. Just one or a few units (such as a medical group or a hospital) can behave as "free riders," in that they continue to receive compensation from the system without committing to increasing the efficiency of their operations. Finally, vertically integrated systems are capital and human resource intensive. Immense capital is required to acquire and maintain the facilities that they own. And with ownership comes the need for staffing and all the attendant problems of maintaining a large cadre of employees: ongoing resolution of union issues; the costs of employee benefits, including health benefits for retirees; turnover; etc. The decision by FHP International Corporation to move out of the staff-model HMO business and to sell its four hospitals is consistent with our perspective that tightly integrated managed care models are no longer competitive.

Organizational Challenges for Virtually Integrated Systems

Virtual integration is not without its challenges. In the long run, the elimination of excess capacity in the market, coupled with the "report card" movement, will require virtually integrated systems to go beyond focusing on reducing units of care and costs per unit. These systems will need to channel their data capabilities into more innovative payment and network arrangements that both lower costs and generate better outcomes. Whatever the panoply of arrangements that evolve, long-term contracting providers with significant patient volume can still leverage patient loyalties in negotiating payment and network conditions.

The negotiation process is also expensive. The downside of contracting is the energy required to negotiate new contracts, renew old ones, and maintain positive working relationships with partners in existing agreements. The onus is on the payer to keep abreast of multiple, dynamic local markets, which requires very effective information management and data analysis to negotiate the most favorable individual contracts.

The bottom line may be that contractual relationships are business relationships, not partnerships, except in the most appealing sense of the word. Contractees are still concerned with individual gain (the degree to which depends on the reimbursement method). Thus, they may have multiple contracts with varying degrees of loyalty to any one payer. The new breed of students choosing medical careers will mitigate this tendency. Today's students and tomorrow's doctors understand at the outset the different demands of a managed care environment and are sensitized to the need for a cost-effective delivery system. This understanding will translate into behavioral changes that are likely to remain more consistent across HMO and insurer contracts.

Provider-Sponsored Networks (PSNs)

The newest forms of IDSs are hospital systems, physician organizations (POs), and physician hospital organizations. Much has been written previously about PHOs because of the concessions that had been sought for such networks under Medicare reform efforts. Because PHOs are also the fastest growing forms of vertically integrated delivery systems, Ernst & Young undertook a survey on physician-hospital integration in 1994 to learn more about this population.[5]

The findings confirmed not only the inherent contradiction in the way PHOs are organized but also the challenges of attempting to merge physicians and hospital cultures faced by most PSNs. Current trends favor movement of health care delivery outside the hospital and away from the overemphasis on acute care and toward an emphasis on primary care providers. PHOs, according to Barry Scheur, President of Scheur Management group, "combin[e] the prices and services of a non-competitive hospital with panicked specialists."[10] PHOs and other provider-sponsored networks fall prey to the trap that integration is an end in itself, not a means for improving system performance.[1]

A number of findings from the Ernst & Young survey, in particular, not only question the long-term viability of PHOs and other PSNs in fiercely competitive managed care markets, but illustrate in bold relief how such entities are subjected to an internal political process that precludes rationalizing delivery. The survey found that most PHOs are, in fact, hospital-initiated. Hospitals are understandably trying to position themselves for managed care, but it may be difficult to avoid tension with health care providers who also desire to control managed care contracting. If the balance of power between physicians and hospital administrators cannot be worked out, the PHO will be undermined.

Provider-sponsored networks must also resist filling empty beds. Intellectually, most hospitals know they have become "cost centers," but some hospitals continue strategies to increase utilization rather than focus on improving their efficiency and organization. Many hospital-sponsored networks also face a limited ability to provide purchasers or payers with broad geographical access, because they are built around single hospitals. Payers are consolidating to cover more markets, and provider-sponsored networks that help them achieve that goal will win contracts.

Ernst & Young also found that most PHOs are specialist-dominated, at a time when payers are more likely to seek provider networks with a higher ratio of primary care physicians (PCPs) to specialists. PHOs may have a hard time offering payers such techniques as primary care case management and an ability to keep inpatient and specialist referral to appropriate levels. Specialists may be particularly resistant to implementing strong utilization management methods, which are necessary for identifying and excluding high-cost, inefficient providers, because of collegial relationships. In some PHOs, the bylaws are written to protect physicians from exclusion and state that physicians may only be terminated for substandard care, not economic reasons.[11] Managed care, however, relies on selective, not inclusive, networks.

A surprising finding in the Ernst & Young survey was that a majority of PHOs have no full-time staff for utilization management, finance, or information systems.

Without a means of knowing and getting a handle on their costs, PSNs cannot succeed in capitated environments. Whether networks assume full risk or contract with payers, they must know their costs in order to price their products or services and to identify problematic areas.

PHOs, POs, and other provider-sponsored networks may face a number of future regulatory challenges. Currently, the National Association of Insurance Commissioners (NAIC) is studying how to create a regulatory model that applies uniform standards to all entities that assume financial risk for the provision of services. The results of two antitrust cases in which the Justice Department ruled that two PHOs had been formed in order to fix prices and that the participating physicians remained competitors could increase scrutiny of these entities at all levels, particularly if Congress agrees to ease the antitrust laws as part of Medicare reform.

Identifying these inherent weaknesses, however, does not mean that PHOs and other vertically integrated provider networks do not have the potential for achieving real economies of scale and reducing costs. However, it does mean that it takes more than just changing the structure of an organization to address the need for systems focused on primary care and prevention; it demands management that is willing to make some hard decisions to be competitive.

PHOs can start hospitals and physicians working together, gaining experience with managed care contracting, and learning to handle the assumption of risk.[11] However, PHOs are especially threatened in more advanced markets, because the balance of power resides with the larger health plans and HMOs that dominate the market. Because they are often required to move quickly into capitated arrangements, many PHOs suffer substantial financial losses. The fact is, PHOs, thus far, are not able to garner significant market penetration.

The Vital Importance of Information Systems

Both fully owned and virtually integrated systems depend heavily on the "glue" of information technology to link all the components together. In integrated systems, data need to be "enterprisewide" and patient-centered.[12] In virtually integrated systems, the integrating organization or network "sponsor" is usually a licensed HMO or insurer that has made substantial investments in data systems that support utilization review, quality management, outcomes assessment, and provider profiling down to the group, clinician, and patient levels. These network sponsors also have the capacity to perform electronic data interface functions critical to linking networks to the sponsor and to each other. Integrated delivery systems that affiliate with HMOs or insurers benefit from this financial investment that they have not themselves made. Currently, for instance, hospitals spend only 2-3 percent of their annual operating budgets on information technology, in contrast to insurance companies, which average 6-7 percent.[12]

As managed care entities mature, computerized patient records will be essential for eliminating waste and unnecessary services from the system. Developments in these types of data systems are coming closer to making data available in real time. The significance is that up-to-date information allows these virtually integrated systems to quickly identify outlier behaviors and use the information to help providers bring their practices in line with prevailing practice models intended to reduce practice variation. Providers who ignore established clinical protocols that have proved to lower costs or improve quality will risk having their contracts terminated.

More sophisticated data systems are also important for implementing disease management—a new approach to controlling costs and improving outcomes that emphasizes the disease process. Disease management is still in its infancy. The lack of accurate and complete medical claims and clinical data remains a barrier. Highly sophisticated information systems are needed to track disease management activities by integrating and linking physician interventions, pharmaceutical therapy, and encounter data. In addition, medical electronic data interchange networks are necessary for supplying health care providers with eligibility, coverage, and treatment guideline information. More innovative and well-capitalized health plans with "existing financial relationships and some degree of control over providers, disease-oriented clinical programs, advanced systems and outcomes assessments capabilities, underwriting skills, and large number of lives under management are best positioned to play a major role in disease management.[13]

Information technology is also integral to providing customers with product choice. Successful health plans of the future will invariably have to maintain simultaneous systems that can monitor diverse provider networks and payment arrangements. Capitation is unlikely to be the dominant form of payment across all managed care products. Clearly, at the same time that the market is transitioning to managed care, consumers are voicing their strong views that they want products that allow self-referral and an ability to seek services outside the provider network. Managed care products will continue to evolve in ways that represent hybrids of PPOs, HMOs, and POS.

Capitation

Some will take exception to the view that all organized systems are not destined to converge toward fully capitated systems. To date, the trend to capitation may be overstated, detracting attention away from what is really going on in the marketplace. There is not a national rush to capitation. Clearly, capitation of primary care physicians and multispecialty groups will grow as more managed care markets mature. Some medical groups may also experiment with subcapitation of specialists, especially those that are forming single-specialty groups. However, capitation of hospitals is moving at a slower pace. In addition, provider-sponsored networks are not necessarily fully capitated, but continue to pay specialists according to a fee schedule.

The big surprise in a recent Southern California survey was the relatively small number of hospital capitation contracts. Only 40 percent reported having at least one capitation contract.[14] As long as there is excess capacity, payers will prefer the rate-cutting strategy of negotiating marginal cost hospital per diem rates (and discounted fees for specialists). Payers will be reluctant to guarantee a percentage of the premium dollar when utilization is still declining.

Thus, it is no surprise that the push for capitated contracts—especially multiple-year contracts—often comes from hospitals, not health plans. Capitating too soon would, in effect, lock in a percentage of the premium dollar at a level above actual costs higher than per diems, which continue to move closer to actual costs. Any payment approach that locks in future revenues eliminates incentives for bringing costs down.

Conclusion

In our view, virtually integrated systems are less subject to the vagaries and paralysis of internal politics that characterize tightly integrated systems. Virtually integrated systems use the competition for payer contracts to ensure that the different components of the organized system continually improve their core competencies. This means physicians focus on providing medical care; hospitals focus on inpatient care; and health plans focus on financing, product design, and information technology to link all these components together. Such systems can adjust faster to the shifting combination of consumer preferences, professional bases of knowledge, and the newest technologies.

Vertically integrated systems, particularly PSNs, exhibit some naiveté in calling for the elimination of the middle man—that is, the managed care plan—because, as the foregoing discussion suggests, the health plan does indeed add value to the system. In contrast to virtually integrated health care systems, vertically integrated systems (full ownership and joint venture) often become insulated from the external pulse of the market and internally beholden to routine processes. Such systems can be undermined by the same bureaucratic tendencies that toppled nation-states committed to central planning.

Our analysis has sought to compare and contrast in order to support broader generalizations. The reality is, while systems may choose a predominant approach, they may also experiment with alternatives in certain markets where they find the local demographic and health system characteristics warrant it. Assessing local markets requires some understanding of the inherent strengths and weaknesses associated with these alternatives. Ultimately, because health care is a locally delivered, locally consumed service, some combination of vertical and virtual strategies may be necessary. Virtually integrated systems may need to acquire medical practices, for example, to enter a new market where providers refuse to contract. Vertically integrated systems may need to contract to broaden enrollee choice or to improve access.

References

1. Gillies, R., and others. "Conceptualizing and Measuring Integration: Findings from the Health Systems Integration Study." *Hospital and Health Services Administration* 38(4):467-89, Winter 1993.
2. Sokolov, J. Information from APM, Inc. New York, New York. *Reproduced in Accountable Health Plans and Advanced Integrated Health Systems.* Washington, D.C.: Health Care Advisory Board, 1994.
3. Shortell, S., and others. "The New World of Managed Care: Creating Organized Delivery Systems." *Health Affairs* 13(5):46-64, Winter 1994.
4. *Integrated Delivery Systems: 8 Industry Models.* Chicago, Ill.: Blue Cross Blue Shield Association, 1994.
5. *Market-Driven Health Care Reform: Physician-Hospital Organizations Profile 1995.* Washington, D.C.: Ernst & Young, LLP; Feb. 1995.
6. Goldsmith, J. "The Illusive Logic of Integration." *Health Care Forum Journal* 37(5):26-31, Sept.-Oct. 1994.
7. "Biotech Industry Sheds Traditional Business Model to Build Virtual Company." *PR NewsWire,* May 22, 1995.
8. "New Strategies for Drug Company Profitability." MarketLetter Ltd (a division of Ziff Communications Co.), Feb. 20, 1995.
9. Blackwood, F. "Strategic Alliances Gain Currency." *San Francisco Business Times* 7(51):2A, Aug. 20, 1993.
10. Sardinha, C., and Taulbee, P. "Many PHOs Are Doomed to Failure, Experts Warn." *Managed Care Outlook,* April 22, 1994, pp. 1-4.
11. Azevedo, D. "PHOs: Castles in the Sand?" *Medical Economics* 71(20):71-84, Oct. 24, 1994.
12. Piper, J. "Provider and Payer Integration: The Latest Trends." *1995 Health Network and Alliance Sourcebook.* Washington, D.C.: Faulkner and Gray, Sept. 1994, pp. 4-28.
13. "The HMO Industry 1995-1996." *C.J. Lawrence Healthcare Services Report*, June 1, 1995, p. 21.
14. Perry, A. "Survey Reveals Complex, Competitive Managed Care Market." *Briefs Focus* (Supplement of Healthcare Association of Southern California), March 31, 1993, pp. 1-5.

Leonard D. Schaeffer is Chair and CEO of Blue Cross of California and of WellPoint Health Networks, Inc., Los Angeles. Dana E. McMurtry was formerly Director, Health Policy and Analysis, Blue Cross of California, Los Angeles. She currently is Director, Health Policy Research, The California Endowment, Woodland Hills.

Chapter 10

Capstone View: The Integration Paradigm Shift

by Kimball Austin Miller, MD, MSHA

The health care delivery system is in the midst of a paradigm shift. Enormous advances in medical science, combined with an almost unceasing national economic growth and a high demand for medical services, during the past 100 years have resulted in the emergence of health care as a growth industry. The tradesman, cottage industry model of independent professionals (clinicians) who visit separate autonomous workshops (hospitals and clinics) to provide services to clients (patients) is being forced to change because of incentives and demands of the managed care process.

For most of the past century, the medical care delivery system consisted of professional services that were directly provided or supervised by physicians. Health care facilities, medical services, and health care resources were always independently ordered or directly recommended by physicians. All medical interventions were covered by payers, largely insurance companies, as long as they were perceived to be medically necessary and appropriate by the physician. In the past, most physician and hospital charges were paid without question, provided that they were "customary and reasonable." However, globalization and the resultant need to limit the labor cost per unit of output have caused an increasing demand by purchasers for a change in health care economics. The fee-for-service reimbursement format and provider-controlled health care delivery model are inherently inflationary and not acceptable in the new price conscious environment. These forces have caused the integration paradigm shift in medical practice delivery organizations.

Although the number and size of group practices have been increasing and alliances of different provider types have been developing for several decades, the pace has dramatically accelerated. Integration, alliances, mergers, and related efforts are attempts to secure a strong position to best meet the growing demand for efficient medical care and health care perceived by consumers to be affordable. The ability of physicians and hospitals to practice independently of one another depended very much on the fee-for-service model of reimbursement and on the ability of patients to continuously switch physicians and hospitals at will. As the buyers of health care services gain in their ability to control provider access and to transfer patients from one service delivery grouping to another depending on price, quality, value, and outcome considerations, all types of health care delivery providers must integrate. As price pressures increase, the ability of disjointed medical care delivery economic units to survive is limited, as buyers react to and are attracted to integrated high-value sellers of health care. To thrive in this new environment, physicians, hospitals, managed care intermediaries, managed care organizations, and physician organizations are all moving toward integrated organizations that incorporate financing, medical management, physician and nonphysician provider services, and institutional care under one partnered umbrella.

As stated in earlier chapters, these integrated practice models are the result of a documented rapid shift of a majority of the nation's commercially insured population into managed care health plans (health maintenance organizations and preferred provider organizations) and the imminent transfer of most of the public sector membership (Medicaid and Medicare) into some form of structured managed care plans. Health care futurists now forecast the growth of the health maintenance organization market from the current 65 million membership to more than 100 million at the start of the next decade.

In the millions of words that have been written in the professional and lay media about the shift in health care delivery format, the ubiquitous theme is integration. When any industry is modified by changes in the economic forces of supply and demand, a realignment of alliances and management processes results. Furthermore, when, simultaneous with an alteration in basic economic forces, there is a market value change from negotiated service pricing to commodity service pricing, the effects of are dramatic, disorienting, and disruptive to participants. However, the paradigm shift has occurred, and providers must rapidly learn about these new formats and incorporate them into their practice styles and organizations.

Reengineering processes are usually defined by the axial terms of horizontal and vertical, but they can also be viewed using the reality terms formal and virtual. Formal integration is the development of a health care delivery system that is fully integrated, with the transfer of all assets and management control to the combined entity. All providers, administrators, and staff are employed by this entity, which can use a centralized or decentralized management style. Virtually integrated systems are also fully vertically integrated, but there is limited transfer of assets to a central organization. In health care, a virtual system is a network of companies strategically aligned to develop and effectively deliver a continuum of managed care services, without common ownership or control, in all clinical settings from health maintenance/acute care to rehabilitation/subacute care. Participants in the integrated system are closely contractually bound to one another, allowing for full integration of clinical services and information systems. Each member of the system shares costs and risk. The operational management style is usually decentralized, with coordination to achieve the agreed upon integration goals and objectives.

In health care delivery, the integration process is neither good nor bad; it is not fundamentally right or wrong. It is the result of economic and social priority changes and of a shift in control from unorganized providers to organized, cost-conscious payers. The initial stage of integration is the operational organizing of various provider groups. As described in detail in earlier chapters, examples of functional or operational organizing are provider alliances, partnership health organizations, physician hospital organizations, physician organizations, independent practice associations, and management service organizations. Organizational integration of the provider group and the managed care intermediary (insurance company) can remain at this operational level or can proceed to structural and asset integration of provider groups (see figure below) and insurance companies.

Integration Models

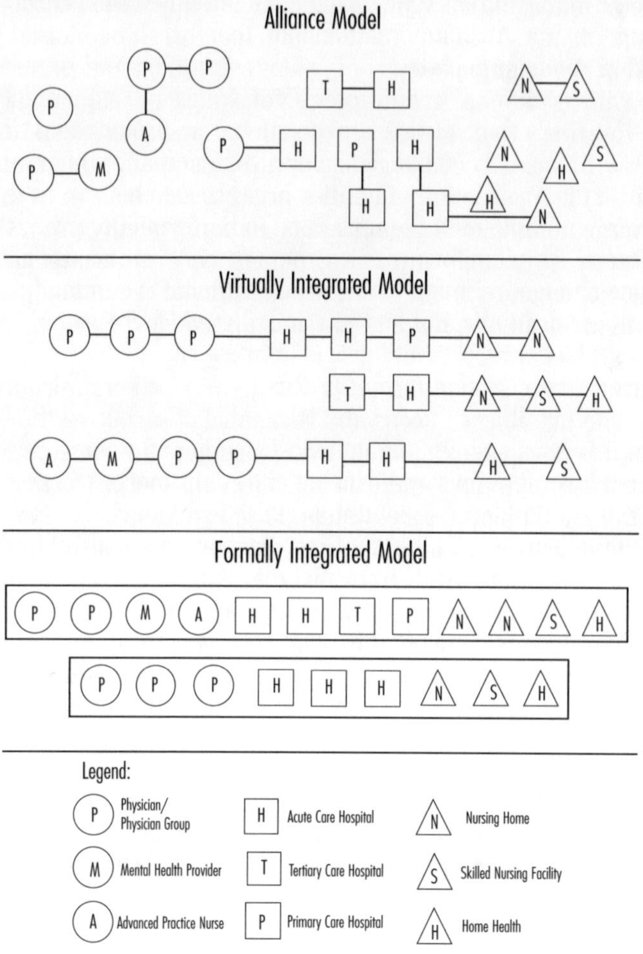

From the organizational management perspective, the full integration process models (formal or virtual) must address the following issues or elements:

- Governance/Control.
- Uniform Operational Process Management.
- Realignment and Reallocation of Resources.
- Maintenance of Quality and Effectiveness.
- Alignment of Insurance Risk and Service Provision.
- Financial/Structural Assets.

Health care providers and their leaders must collaborate with health care administrators to determine the elements of the integration management process model that they are ready, willing, and able to integrate. The process must be built on open communication of management style, organizational objectives, corporate culture, and financial statements. As in any relationship, there must be mutual growth. The usual relationship development steps of forming, storming, and performing, which are consistent with traditional group interaction, must be sequentially addressed and resolved. The first result of this organizational and operational management relationship growth is usually collaboration or a contractually bound integrated system—a system that is a collection of entities organized to behave in the market as if they were a large multifaceted organization. To perform effectively, the members of the system must have uniform clinical patient care protocols, an operational information system, a commitment to reduce operational redundancy, and common financial incentives for all hospital and physician providers.

This health care delivery system format is able to provide services across the total spectrum of patient health care needs and is capable of accepting the financial risk associated with this responsibility. After "living together" for some period, the partners can decide if it is mutually beneficial to "marry" or merge the assets into a formal vertically integrated health care system. Practical knowledge has documented the importance of selectively picking "lifetime" partners because of the financial and psychological problems that result from divorce. Current studies seem to indicate that recent capital investments made by health care organizations to acquire multiple hospitals, physician practices, third-party administration agents, and health plans have high up-front costs and are rarely able to achieve financial investment objectives. Some asset integrated systems are starting the devolution process and changing into virtually integrated networks.

Independent of model type, providers must understand that, to succeed in the current managed care environment, the integrated entity must be able to provide clinical services conveniently and in an efficient format. They must use medical management principles and community health status monitoring to obtain a high patient-perceived value and to fill the needs, wants, and demands of all private and public payers. Clinicians, physician executives, and health system administrators must work collaboratively to eliminate excess costs, improve the quality of patient care, document clinical outcomes, and increase provider productivity. It is important to understand that this represents a major shift from the traditional model of the physician provider and hospital as autonomous entities to the current model, which is collective, collaborative, and risk sharing.

Economic and social forces have caused the health care paradigm shift in medical care delivery. Integration is being proposed as the "brass ring" solution in the current health care marketplace. As physician and hospital providers grasp an organizational design, they must decide either to put the ring on their organizational finger or put it around their waist as a life preserver and just hold hands with the next traveler in the turbulent sea of health care change.

Kimball Austin Miller, MD, MSHA, is Adjunct Professor of Business Administration, Arizona State University, College of Business, Department of Health Administration and Policy, Tempe, Arizona, and Adjunct Associate Professor of Medicine, University of Oklahoma, College of Medicine, Department of Internal Medicine, Tulsa, Oklahoma.

Index

A

accrual, 6
actuarial assumptions, 6
administrative costs, 6
administrative leadership, 69
adverse selection, 6
age/gender factor, 6
ambulatory patient grouping, 6
antitrust, 86

B

balance billing, 6
bed leasing, 29
benefit package, 7
Blue Cross and Blue Shield, 20
budgeting, 42
bundling, 13
business health coalition, 7

C

capitalization, 82
capitation, 7,29,31,134
care management, 34
carve-out, 7
case management, 7
case rates, 28
case review, 37
CHMIS, 7
choice, 55
closed-panel model, 7,24
coinsurance, 7
committees, 85
community health management information system, 7
community rating, 7
competition, 71
concurrent review, 7,36
consolidation, 72
continued stay review, 36
continuity of care, 54
contracts, 83,101
copayment, 8
CPT-4, 8
credentialing, 8,38
Current Procedural Terminology, 8

D

deductible, 8
demand management, 4,8,35
Department of Justice, 86
diagnosis-related group, 8,28
differential by day in hospital, 28
direct contracting option, 8
discounted fee for service, 8

discounts, 27
disease management, 37
DRG, 8,28

E

echo analysis, 8
EDI, 8
electronic data interchange, 8
Employee Retirement Income Security Act, 8,20
enrollment, 48
EPMPY, 8
EPO, 8
ERISA, 8,20
evaluation and management services, 9
exclusive provider organization, 8

F

Federal Trade Commission, 82,86
fee schedule, 9
fee-for-service reimbursement, 9,34
formulary, 9
FTC, 82

G

gatekeeper, 9,35,48,67
gate opener, 9
governance, 81,119
Group Health Association of Washington, 2
Group Health Cooperative of Puget Sound, 2,47
group model, 9

H

HCFA 1500, 9,110
Health Care Financing Administration (HCFA), 9
Health Insurance Plan of New York, 48
health maintenance organization, 9,22
Health Plan Employer Data and Information Set, 9
health plans, types, 20
health risk appraisals, 35
health status questionnaire, 9
HEDIS, 9
HMO, 9,22
HMO Act of 1973, 1,49
HMO-affiliated MSO, 93
HMO models, 5
horizontal integration, 10
hospital perspective, 56
hospital reimbursement, 26
hospital role in PHO, 78
hospital-sponsored MSO, 93

I

IBNR, 42
ICD-9-CM, 10
IDS, 10

incentive payments, 31
incurred but not reported, 42
indemnity insurance, 21
indemnity plan, 10
independent practice association, 10,63
information systems, 83,133
integrated health care system, 10,67, 113,125,137
integrated service network, 10
integration models, 128,139
investor-sponsored MSO, 93
IPA, 10
ISN, 10

J

Joint Commission for Accreditation of Healthcare Organizations (JCAHO), 10,38

K

Kaiser, Henry, 47
Kaiser-Permanente Medical Care, 2

L

large-case management, 37
legal issues, 86
local competition, 71
loss ratio, 10

M

managed care enrollment, 48
managed care growth, 18
managed care intermediary, 10
managed care organization, 10
management information system, 11
management service organization, 92
market evolution, 126
married, 13,66
Mayo Clinic, 48
MCI, 10
MCO, 10
medical loss ratio, 10
medical management, 4
Medicare, 52
mental health services, 55
MIS, 11
mixed model, 25
models of managed care, 65
MSO, 92

N

National Committee on Quality Assurance (NCQA), 11
network model, 11,25
nonparticipating physician, 11

O

open-access HMOs, 23
open-format model, 11
open-panel plans, 24
outcome measure, 11
outcomes, 58
outpatient procedures, 30

P

package pricing, 28
paradigm shift, 138
participating physician, 11
patient perspective, 55
pattern analysis, 37
PCN, 11
PCP, 11
pediatric care, 54
peer review, 11
penalties, 30
per diem reimbursement, 11
per member per month, 11,29,40
per member per year, 42
per thousand members per year, 42
pharmacoeconomics, 11
PHO, 11,75,131
PHO committees, 85
PHO contracts, 83
PHO funding, 83
PHO governance, 81
physician compensation, 30
physician/hospital joint venture MSO, 93
physician hospital organization, 11,75, 131
physician organization, 12,79,108,131
physician role in PHO, 79
PMPM, 11,29,40
PMPY, 42
PO, 12,79,108,131
point of service, 12,25
POS, 12,25
PPO, 12,22
practice guidelines, 12
preferred provider organization, 12,22
premium rate development, 42
preventive care, 52
primary care network, 11
primary care provider, 11
primary specialist provider, 12
prior authorization, 12
prospective review, 35
provider, 12
provider perspective, 56
provider reimbursement, 25,30,105
provider services agreement, 110
provider-sponsored network, 131
PSN, 131
PSP, 12

Q

QRC, 109
quality assurance, 12
quality management, 38
quality review, 109
quality review committee, 109

R

RBRVS, 13
reengineering, 138
referral services, 35
regional competition, 71
reinsurance, 12
relationship management, 12
relative value unit, 12
resource-based relative value scale, 13
resource management, 44
retrospective review, 37
risk, 3,2243,76
risk assumption, 43
risk contracting, 101

S

self-funded plans, 20
self-insured plan, 13
service plan, 20
service-related case rates, 28
sliding scale discount on charges, 27
sliding scale per diem, 28
staff model, 13
"Statements of Antitrust Enforcement Policy in Healthcare," 86
stop loss, 13
straight charges, 27
straight discount on charges, 27
straight per diem charges, 27
system governance, 119

T

telemedicine, 13
third-party administrator, 13,20
total quality management, 13
TPA, 13,20
TQM, 13
trust, 78

U

UB-92, 13
UCR, 13
UMC, 107
unbundling, 13
unmarried, 13,66
utilization, 52
utilization management, 14,34,107
utilization management committee, 107
utilization review, 14

V

value, 14
vertical integration, 14,113,125
virtual integration, 129

W

withholds, 14,30